ABC of
Autism

ABC of

Autism

Munib Haroon

Consultant Community Paediatrician
Harrogate and District NHS Foundation Trust
Harrogate, UK

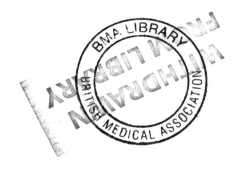

WILEY Blackwell

Registered Office(s)
John Wiley & Sons, Inc., 111 River Street, Hoboken, NJ 07030, USA
John Wiley & Sons Ltd, The Atrium, Southern Gate, Chichester, West Sussex, PO19 8SQ, UK

Editorial Office
9600 Garsington Road, Oxford, OX4 2DQ, UK

For details of our global editorial offices, customer services, and more information about Wiley products visit us at www.wiley.com.

Wiley also publishes its books in a variety of electronic formats and by print-on-demand. Some content that appears in standard print versions of this book may not be available in other formats.

Library of Congress Cataloging-in-Publication Data

Names: Haroon, Munib, author.
Title: ABC of autism / Munib Haroon.
Description: Hoboken, NJ : Wiley-Blackwell, 2019. |Series: ABC series | Includes bibliographical references and index. |
Identifiers: LCCN 2018060333 (print) | LCCN 2018060681 (ebook) | ISBN 9781119317272 (Adobe PDF) |
    ISBN 9781119317227 (ePub) | ISBN 9781119317258 (pbk.)
Subjects: | MESH: Autism Spectrum Disorder–diagnosis |Autism Spectrum Disorder–therapy
Classification: LCC RC553.A88 (ebook) | LCC RC553.A88(print) | NLM WS 350.8.P4 | DDC616.85/882–dc23
LC record available at https://lccn.loc.gov/2018060333

Cover Design: Wiley
Cover Image: © DrAfter123/Getty Images

Set in 9.25/12pt Minion by SPi Global, Pondicherry, India
Printed and bound in Singapore by Markono Print Media Pte Ltd

10 9 8 7 6 5 4 3 2 1

Contents

Contributors

Dr Ruth Bevan

Consultant in Gender Dysphoria
Northern Region Gender Dysphoria Service
Newcastle, UK

Dr Kate Cooper

Clinical Psychologist/Honorary Lecturer
University of Bath
Bath, UK

Dr Conor Davidson

Consultant Psychiatrist
Leeds Autism Diagnostic Service
Leeds, UK

Ms Isabelle Gately

Teacher
Elizabeth Garrett Anderson School
London, UK

Dr Derek Glidden

Consultant Psychiatrist
Nottingham Centre for Transgender Health
and Nottingham City Asperger Service
Nottingham, UK

Dr Munib Haroon

Consultant Community Paediatrician
Harrogate and District NHS Foundation Trust
Harrogate, UK

Dr Alwyn Kam

Specialty Doctor in Psychiatry of Learning Disability
Leeds Autism Diagnostic Service (LADS)
Leeds, UK

Dr Keri-Michele Lodge

Specialty Registrar Psychiatry of Intellectual Disability
Leeds Autism Diagnostic Service
Leeds, UK

Ms Frances Needham

Former Clinical Team Manager, Neurodevelopmental Service
Leeds Autism Diagnostic Service
Leeds, UK

Dr Mini G. Pillay

Consultant Child and Adolescent Psychiatrist (Learning Disabilities)
Wakefield CAMHS
Wakefield, UK

Dr Padakkara Saju

Consultant Psychiatrist
Leeds Gender Identity Services
Leeds, UK

Dr Monica Shaha

Consultant in Child and Adolescent Psychiatry
Psychiatry-UK LLP
Dewsbury, UK

Dr Alison Stansfield

Consultant Psychiatrist and Clinical Lead
Leeds Autism Diagnostic Service
Leeds, UK

Acknowledgements

I would like to thank all of the chapter contributors for giving up their valuable time, sharing their expertise and insights, not minding my endless tinkering and, on one occasion, reviewing drafts and responding to me whilst they were on holiday (AS). A big thank you therefore should also go to their nearest and dearest, as the opportunity cost of writing a book is often time away from family and loved ones.

All of us have benefitted from having patients, carers, mentors, colleagues, friends and acquaintances (Aspies and Neurotypicals) who are a source of inspiration, advice and learning. It is to be hoped that this book benefits from their collective wisdom in a similar manner.

I would like to thank the editorial team at Wiley, especially James Watson, Commissioning Editor, and Yogalakshmi Mohanakrisnan, Project Editor, who have helped midwife the book from conception, through an elephantine gestational period, to delivery. Their expert advice was invaluable, and that telephone call before the very last 'push' greatly reassuring.

A number of people read chapters and provided thoughtful comments: Clare Armstrong-Roger, Lynn Drinkwater, Anu Raykundalia, Bob Phillips – thank you. Other colleagues and friends have been there to listen, to offer their thoughts, to give their insights and encouragement, and I thank you all.

Finally, to Sophie, who has put up with, and supported, the Sisyphean task of writing and editing this book – and a lot more besides – thank you! This is for you.

Munib Haroon
3 August 2018
Harrogate, UK

Abbreviations

ADHD	attention deficit hyperactivity disorder
ADI-R	Autism Diagnostic Interview – Revised
ADOS	Autism Diagnostic Observation Schedule
AMAB/AFAB	assigned male at birth/assigned female at birth
ASC	autism spectrum condition
ASD	autism spectrum disorder
ASDI	Asperger Syndrome (and high-functioning autism) Diagnostic Interview
ASSQ	Autism Spectrum Screening Questionnaire
BNF	*British National Formulary*
CAMHS	Child and Adolescent Mental Health Services
CAST	Childhood Autism Spectrum Test
CBT	cognitive behavioural therapy
CGH	Comparative Genomic Hybridisation
CI	confidence interval
CNV	copy number variation
3Di	Developmental, Dimensional and Diagnostic Interview
DISCO	Diagnostic Interview for Social and Communication Disorders
DSM	Diagnostic and Statistical Manual
DVLA	Driver and Vehicle Licensing Agency
EHCP	Education, Health and Care Plan
GARS	Gilliam Autism Rating Scale
GV	gender variance
ICD	International Classification of Disease
ID	intellectual disability
IEP	Individual Education Plan
LADS	Leeds Autism Diagnostic Service
LD	learning disability
MMR	measles, mumps, and rubella
NICE	National Institute for Health and Clinical Excellence
OCD	obsessive compulsive disorder
OR	odds ratio
PD	personality disorder
PDA	pathological demand avoidance
PDD-NOS	pervasive developmental disorder not otherwise specified
PECS	Picture Exchange Communication System
RAADS-R	Ritvo Autism Asperger Diagnostic Scale – Revised
SENCO	Special Educational Needs Coordinator
SIGN	Scottish Intercollegiate Guidelines Network
SMART	Specific, Measurable, Achievable, Realistic, Timely
SNP	single nucleotide polymorphism
SSRI	selective serotonin reuptake inhibitor
STOMP	Stopping Over-Medication of People
TEACCH	Treatment and Education of Autistic and related Communication handicapped Children
WHO	World Health Organization

CHAPTER 1

An Introduction to Autism

Munib Haroon

OVERVIEW

- Autism is a relatively common neurodevelopmental condition with a prevalence of over 1% in many populations.
- Autism is defined by the presence of social communication and social interaction difficulties and restricted, repetitive patterns of behaviour, interests and activities which can vary in severity.
- Autism has a heterogeneous clinical presentation because of variations in the core features and the presence or absence of associated conditions.
- The diagnosis of autism is a clinical diagnosis.
- There is no cure for autism but early intervention can have a significant impact upon overall well-being.

Definition

Autism spectrum disorder (or autism) is a relatively common neurodevelopmental condition with a heterogeneous underlying basis which is incompletely understood. The definition of autism is based on the presence of impairments in social communication and social interaction and restricted, repetitive patterns of behaviour, interests or activities (Figure 1.1). These impairments vary greatly in severity, and whilst often noticeable during childhood can go undetected until later in life.

The neurodiversity movement has had a large impact on the terms of discourse when referring to autism and, for many people, use of the term 'autism spectrum condition' is preferred to the use of the term '… disorder', whilst plural terminology (e.g. 'disorders') is also often used to highlight the heterogeneous nature of the condition. The terms 'autism,' 'autism spectrum disorder(s)' and, occasionally, 'autism spectrum condition', are therefore used interchangeably in this book. (However, for diagnostic purposes, in a clinical setting, it remains sensible to use conventional terminology in a consistent way to avoid confusion.)

History

The term 'autism' is derived from the Greek word 'autos,' meaning 'self,' and was first used in 1910 by Eugen Bleuler (Figure 1.2) in relation to schizophrenia, to describe the withdrawal of schizophrenic patients into their own fantasies. However, the earliest clinically based descriptions of what we would now recognise to be autistic patients were not written until many years later (although there is considerable interest amongst researchers in older historical descriptions of individuals who seem to possess autistic traits). The first well-described clinical account was written by Sukhareva in 1926 although credit for the first detailed descriptions of autism are usually attributed to Leo Kanner in 1943 and then to Hans Asperger in 1944. Opinion is divided over who 'got there first', and who knew what about the other's work – a controversial area which lies outside the scope of this book. Asperger's seminal contribution to the field fell into neglect in the years around the Second World War before being rehabilitated in 1981 by Lorna Wing who coined the eponymous term 'Asperger's syndrome'.

Epidemiology

The reported prevalence of autism has increased in recent decades, with estimates of over 1% being made in some large-scale surveys. It is not yet clear how much of this increase could be caused by an actual increased incidence or whether it is just that the change is the result of better public awareness, improved recognition by professionals and a widening of the diagnostic criteria.

Large-scale studies have shown that autism affects 2–3 times more males than females. This could be because of under-recognition in females or because of a genuine sex difference.

Aetiology

Controversy over aetiology has dogged the condition from early on. It was seen – erroneously – by some as an acquired condition resulting from parent–child interactions, with 'blame' in some quarters

---

ABC of Autism, First Edition. Munib Haroon.

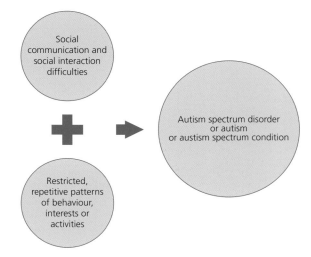

Figure 1.1 Autism is defined by the presence of features in two broad categories.

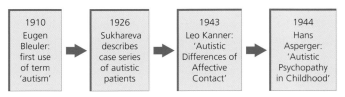

Figure 1.2 A timeline involving some of the early pioneers in autism.

attached to 'refrigerator mums' – a theory that was popularised in the 1950s by Bruno Bettelheim. The 1960s saw a shift from 'nurture-based' explanatory models towards 'nature-based' models and towards undertaking research to address the biological basis for the disease. This biological basis remains incompletely understood. What is clear is that there is a strong genetic basis for autism, along with a clear role for environmental risk factors. It has been known for some time that a sibling of an affected individual is more likely to have autism than a general member of the population: 10% in comparison to 1%. Furthermore, the risk of a monozygotic twin having autism is greater than the risk in a dizygotic twin. More recent research has identified that there are multiple candidate genetic mutations, many of which are uncommon or rare, whose interactions may have a role in how the autistic phenotype is expressed. It is thought that the non-genetic risk factors that have been identified may interact with genetic factors and thus affect how a phenotype is expressed in an individual. Some of this work has not been without controversy, most notably the well-publicised scare over a study (published and subsequently retracted by *The Lancet*) that erroneously showed an association between the mumps, measles and rubella (MMR) vaccine and autism and which led to a significant decline in immunisation rates in the UK in the early 21st century.

Clinical features

Whilst the origin of the term 'autism' suggests a person's withdrawal into themselves, the idea that everyone with autism is highly withdrawn and isolated is incorrect and only describes a

proportion of individuals with the condition. The term 'spectrum' is used to denote the heterogeneity that is seen in the clinical features of different individuals with the condition. In addition, the autistic phenotype is often expressed differently within the same individual as they move from childhood to adolescence and adulthood.

As well as the core features, those with autism can present with co-morbid or associated conditions: mood disorders, anxiety disorders, attention deficit hyperactivity disorder (ADHD), learning disability, dyspraxia and epilepsy.

Diagnosis

The diagnosis of autism can theoretically be made at any age, although it would take confidence to make a diagnosis in a child below the age of 2–3 years. The mean age of diagnosis in the UK is currently about 5 years although a diagnosis can occur several decades after this. Such a late diagnosis occurs in many contexts: where the presentation is subtle and associated with normal IQ and speech, in looked-after children, or where there is a significant learning disability or other co-morbidity making recognition of the underlying autistic features difficult.

A diagnosis is made based on clinical assessment including history (including developmental and psychiatric information), examination, observations from other parties and, sometimes, the use of diagnostic clinical examination tools. At present there is no role for blood tests or imaging to make a diagnosis although they may help to diagnose associated or underlying conditions.

Management

The core features of autism cannot be cured or removed with treatment. However, support, particularly early intervention, can have positive effects, whilst co-morbidities are amenable to treatment if recognised. Medication can, in the right circumstances, be used to manage many associated medical problems and co-morbidities: sleep difficulties, ADHD, aggression, mood disorders and anxiety.

Prognosis and outcome

A normal trajectory for the development of childhood communication skills and normal IQ seem to be good predictors for later outcome. The presence of associated co-morbidities is likely to have a significant effect on how a person with autism manages in life and so the early identification and management of these, if and when they arise, is important. Non-biological factors such as the nearby presence of friends and family and the ability to take part in some sort of social activities can also be very important – and, importantly, more malleable than biological factors.

It is increasingly recognised that individuals with autism are at an increased risk of early mortality due to epilepsy, and suicide (because of psychiatric illness), whilst those with significant levels of social communication difficulty and cognitive impairment can struggle with many aspects of day-to-day life including school,

Box 1.1 **Outcomes for autism**

- Less than 20% of adults with autism have a full-time job
- Less than 20% of adults with autism live independently
- Less than 30% of adults with autism have a driving licence
- On average, people with autism die 16 years earlier than the general population
- Individuals with autism and a learning disability die, on average, 30 years earlier than the general population

employment, long-term relationships and independent living (Box 1.1). But, at the same time, many people with autism lead rich, fulfilling, independent or semi-independent lives whilst making valuable contributions to society. Every person with autism – like every person without autism – is a unique individual and should be treated as such.

Further reading

American Psychiatric Association. Diagnostic and Statistical Manual of Mental Disorders, 5th edn. Washington DC: American Psychiatric Association, 2013.

Brett D, Warnell F, McConachie H, Parr J. Factors affecting age at ASD diagnosis in UK: no evidence that diagnosis age has decreased between 2004 and 2014. Journal of Autism and Developmental Disorders 2016; 46: 1974–1984.

Kuhn R. Eugen Bleuler's concepts of psychopathology. History of Psychiatry 2004; 15: 361–366.

Lai MC, Lombardo MV, Baron-Cohen S. Autism. Lancet 2014; 383: 896–910.

Manouilenko I, Bejerot S. Sukhareva: prior to Asperger and Kanner. Nordic Journal of Psychiatry 2015; 69: 479–482.

Scottish Intercollegiate Guidelines Network (SIGN). SIGN 145: assessment, diagnosis and interventions for autism spectrum disorders. Edinburgh: SIGN, 2016. Available from: https://www.sign.ac.uk/assets/sign145.pdf. Accessed 15 November 2018.

Volkmar F, Wolf J. When children with autism become adults. World Psychiatry 2013; 12: 79–80.

Wolf S. The history of autism. European Child and Adolescent Psychiatry 2004; 13: 201–208.

CHAPTER 2

Classification and Diagnosis

Munib Haroon

OVERVIEW

- Good classification systems for diseases and conditions are important for diagnosis and research and to enable consistent and clear communication among professionals, patients and carers.
- There are two main classification systems for autism spectrum disorders: DSM and ICD.
- DSM-5 is the most recently updated classification system.
- The term 'autism spectrum disorder' is an umbrella term for conditions like Asperger's syndrome.

Classification systems of disease and illness are an important tool in modern health care for several reasons. They are the foundation upon which a standardised diagnostic process can be established, and they are the basis for making and communicating evidence-based judgements and decisions about treatment and prognosis. Having a consistent way of talking about a condition benefits not only the doctor–patient relationship, but also allows for data to be organised and collected in a systematic fashion which can then be put to epidemiological use and for clinical research. To put it another way, it is important that when a person says that particular individuals or a group have 'autism' everyone else – including doctors, patients, parents, researchers, commissioners and those making public health decisions – can understand and be completely clear what 'autism' means and on what basis this decision has been made.

However, there are a few challenges with the classification and diagnosis of autism although these challenges are not unique to this condition. First, autism can probably be thought of as a number of disorders that have features in common, and so a useful classification needs to be broad enough to take this variation into account. Then there is the problem of a lack of sensitive and specific biomarkers (e.g. genetic or radiological or other biological 'diagnostic' tests) which can help us to say that a particular patient has autism. As a result, autism spectrum disorders, like a number of other neurodevelopmental disorders, are behaviourally defined conditions.

This leads to the question of what is 'normal' and what is 'abnormal'. These kinds of distinctions are difficult to make with behaviour, because it does not exist in a binary state but comes in 'shades of grey'. A related challenge is recognising the abnormal but then determining the exact nature of the abnormality – for example, is this abnormality 'mania' or it is 'hyperactivity' and how are these individual features themselves classified (let alone an entire disorder)?

This is an ongoing debate and a challenge for a few areas in medicine. Part of the solution may lie in the identification of biomarkers for autism (if they can be developed) and for diagnostic and classification systems to map better onto our developing understanding of how the brain functions.

Having noted all of this we can think about what might make a good classification system and this is outlined in Box 2.1.

The practical difficulty with having different classifications, especially those that look at behaviourally defined conditions is that: (i) the terminology within one classification system can change from one edition to the next; and (ii) the terminology in different classification systems can vary at any one point in time.

For clinicians and researchers this poses a number of questions such as, 'Which is the best classification for us to use?' and 'Does moving from one scheme to the next (or from one iteration to the next) affect how we make a diagnosis?' and finally 'Does using new terminology affect previous diagnoses that we have made?'

All of this is probably an argument for having fewer rather than more classifications, having more standardised terminology, investigating the role of biomarkers in classification and diagnosis, and more co-operation between those who develop these schemes.

Current classification schemes

Over time, several classifications schemes for autism and related disorders have been proposed, but the two most widely used are the American Psychiatric Association's Diagnostic and Statistical Manual (DSM) which is now into its fifth edition (DSM-5) and the World Health Organization's (WHO) International Classification of Disease which is currently in its tenth iteration (ICD-10) with the eleventh planned for publication in 2018.

DSM-5

Used widely in the USA (but also in Europe, including in the UK), and updated in 2013, the DSM-5 classification uses the overarching term of 'autism spectrum disorder' instead of the terminology from previous editions of the DSM – 'pervasive developmental disorders'. This single term now replaces the older subclassifications (e.g. 'autism', 'Asperger's syndrome' 'pervasive developmental disorders not otherwise specified' PDD-NOS) with the aim of allowing for more consistent use of terminology by clinicians and researchers, but with the idea that someone previously diagnosed with Asperger's syndrome would be considered in the newer classification to have an autism spectrum disorder (Figure 2.1). The concept of the clinical heterogeneity seen in autism is represented not only in the use of the term 'spectrum', but also in the use of specifiers that indicate severity and associated features.

In addition to these changes, the concept of autism as a condition whose core features exist as a 'triad of impairments' (social interaction difficulties; social communication difficulties; restricted, repetitive patterns of behaviour, interests or activities) has been re-termed as a dyad by merging the first two components into social communication and social interaction difficulties because of the recognition that the two components are inextricably interlinked (Figure 2.2).

For those who have social difficulties without the restricted, repetitive behavioural elements, a separate criterion for 'social communication disorder' has been developed under which such individuals should be considered, and this incorporates some of those who would previously have fallen under the PDD-NOS term.

According to the classification, a diagnosis is made in the presence of sufficient features affecting the dyad, and which affect function and are severe enough to require support (or substantial or very substantial support) and whose features have been present since early developmental life (although these may be masked by learned strategies or intellectualisation or may not become apparent until demands exceed native ability) and are not better explained by intellectual disability or global developmental delay. Once a diagnosis is made, DSM allows for a number of modifiers to be made to a standalone diagnosis of autism spectrum disorder. This includes intellectual and language impairments and the presence of other medical, genetic, neurodevelopmental, psychiatric or behavioural conditions (Figure 2.2).

ICD-10

The ICD-10 uses the overarching term 'pervasive developmental disorders' which includes the conditions 'childhood autism', 'atypical autism' and 'Asperger's syndrome'. It uses the concept of abnormalities or impairments involving a triad. However, ICD-11 is likely to see this change, with similar overarching terminology being used, like DSM-5, to describe someone as having an 'autism spectrum disorder' as well as a move away from the triad to the dyad.

What does a clinician use? DSM or ICD?

For autism spectrum disorders, both the UK National Institute for Health and Clinical Excellence (NICE) and Scottish Intercollegiate Guidelines Network (SIGN) refer clinicians in the UK to either DSM or ICD. It is important that whichever scheme is used that it is the most recent version and that it is used in a consistent manner rather than a mix and match approach. In this regard, it is important to consider how this is done within a department to enable clear and consistent communication with patients, families and

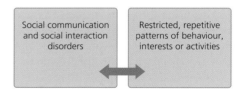

Figure 2.2 The DSM-5 classification of autism spectrum disorder is based on the presence of features affecting the dyad since early on in development, and which are clinically significant and for which there is no better explanation. The scheme allows for each element of the dyad to be 'graded' for severity and for specifiers to be attached to the diagnosis.

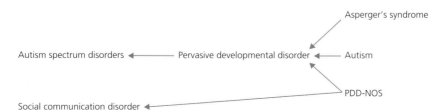

Figure 2.1 In DSM-5, the term 'autism spectrum disorder' has replaced older terms such as 'pervasive developmental disorder' and 'Asperger's syndrome'.

other professionals. This book has opted to use the DSM-5 classification primarily because it has become increasingly used worldwide, including in the UK, and because at the time of writing it was the most up-to-date of the two classification schemes.

Asperger's syndrome

The term Asperger's syndrome has been 'swallowed-up' in DSM-5 by the overarching term 'autism spectrum disorder' (and so is no longer used by that classification) with the implication that it is one of a type of these disorders. Asperger's syndrome in simple terms was defined as a disorder in which many of the core features of autism were present but where *clinically significant* difficulties with language delay, cognition, self-help or adaptive skills were not part of the picture. The previous separation between autism and Asperger's syndrome as diagnostic entities, and the presence of several different diagnostic criteria for Asperger's, had the potential to create difficulties, including how to decide whether someone had autism *or* Asperger's when it was hard to define strictly what a clinically significant difficulty was. There was also the potential for problems with the consistent use of the term in different settings. As such, use of the more overarching term alone is seen as helpful for both clinical and research reasons. However, there are a few difficulties with this approach. First, many individuals strongly identify with the term Asperger's syndrome (and use the self-referential term 'Aspie'), and may see themselves as distinct from the 'general' autistic phenotype. Secondly, it has been felt that the term 'Asperger' may have less stigma attached to it and thus there might be benefits in using the term in some instances. Thirdly, the term, by virtue of being more narrow when applied correctly to certain individuals, has been considered a better descriptor than just saying that a person has 'autism'. At the time of writing, in 2018, although the ICD-11 has not yet been released, many units are choosing to use the overarching term 'autism spectrum disorder' instead of making a diagnosis of Asperger's syndrome when it might have been appropriate to do so in the past. (This book will use autism spectrum disorder instead of Asperger's syndrome.)

Pathological demand avoidance

In recent years there has been considerable interest in the term 'pathological demand avoidance' (PDA) and its use as a separate diagnosis or as a co-diagnosis alongside that of autism. Whilst it is used by some to describe a range of complex behaviours seen in individuals with autism (and possibly without autism), it is not identified in DSM-5 as an independent syndrome.

It is likely that the term fits a constellation of co-occurring features in autistic people where the presentation is also shaped by certain social, familial and mental health factors (such as the presence of coexisting anxiety disorders, ADHD and oppositional defiance disorder).

Further reading

American Psychiatric Association. Diagnostic and Statistical Manual of Mental Disorders (fifth edn.). Washington, DC: American Psychiatric Publishing, 2013.

Baird G, Norbury CF. Social (pragmatic) communication disorders and autism spectrum disorder. Archives of Disease in Childhood 2016; 101: 745–751.

Gillberg C. A Guide to Asperger Syndrome. Cambridge: Cambridge University Press, 2002.

Green J, Absoud M, Grahame V, et al. Pathological Demand Avoidance: symptoms but not a syndrome. Lancet Child and Adolescent Health 2018; 2: 455–464.

World Health Organization. The ICD-10 Classification of Mental and Behavioural Disorders: Clinical Descriptions and Diagnostic Guidelines. Geneva: World Health Organization, 1992.

CHAPTER 3

The Aetiology of Autism

Keri-Michele Lodge

OVERVIEW

- The aetiology of autism spectrum disorder (ASD) is incompletely understood.
- Current evidence suggests ASD is a multifactorial disorder resulting from a complex interplay between genetic and environmental factors.
- Uncommonly, ASD can be a presenting feature of a specific genetic syndrome.
- There is no link between the measles, mumps and rubella (MMR) vaccine and ASD.

The aetiology of autism spectrum disorder (ASD) is incompletely understood and continuously evolving. As such, this chapter provides an overview of the topic.

As well as being a clinically heterogeneous disorder, autism is also aetiologically heterogeneous – autism is not a single condition with a single cause. Instead, current research suggests that ASD is a multifactorial disorder arising from a complex interplay between genetic and environmental factors that impact upon neurodevelopment (Figure 3.1). As well as genetic features that confer susceptibility upon individuals, it is postulated that environmental factors influence whether those with a genetic predisposition develop ASD. In addition, epigenetic factors that alter gene expression without changing the primary gene sequence are thought to play an important part, and are themselves influenced by environmental factors. The precise genetic, epigenetic and environmental factors involved in the aetiology of ASD are yet to be fully defined. Similarly, the mechanism by which these factors interact and lead to abnormalities in neurodevelopment, and how these in turn affect brain function, are subjects of ongoing research.

Genetic factors

ASD has a strong genetic basis. ASD aggregates in families, and the heritability is high. The risk of having ASD increases with increasing genetic relatedness. Children born in families where a sibling already has ASD have a much greater risk of having ASD. In dizygotic twins, the probability of one twin having ASD if the other is affected is in the order of around 10%. In monozygotic twins, studies suggest this figure may be as high as 82–92%. In addition, first degree relatives of people with ASD have an increased chance of having features associated with ASD without meeting the diagnostic criteria for ASD (known as 'subthreshold traits', or the 'broader autistic phenotype'), such as mild deficits in social understanding and mild language dysfunction.

ASD can occur in association with syndromes that have defined genetic causes, for example, fragile X syndrome, tuberous sclerosis and Smith–Lemli–Opitz syndrome. However, such conditions are rare, and together account for only around 5–15% of cases of ASD.

The genetics of ASD is complicated. In most people with ASD, there is no identifiable genetic cause. Highly penetrant single gene mutations (Box 3.1) exist but may account for a minority of cases of ASD. Most cases are probably a result of relatively common genetic variations that individually confer only a small elevation in risk but which, when present together in sufficient numbers in an individual, can interact together to cause ASD. In some cases, de novo genetic mutations underlie the development of ASD, whilst the reported link between increased paternal age and increased risk of ASD may be a consequence of the presence of germline mutations in the offspring of older fathers. Research into both advancing paternal and maternal age and the risk of ASD is ongoing.

Studies have looked at the association between autism and genetic variations including chromosomal abnormalities, copy number variations (CNVs), single-nucleotide polymorphisms (SNPs) and other mutations involving candidate genes. To date, hundreds of candidate genes have been implicated, with studies suggesting many loci for ASD susceptibility genes (Table 3.1). However, a recent meta-analysis of candidate gene association studies concluded that previous studies have been underpowered, highlighting the need for further studies with larger sample sizes to identify which common variants of possible candidate genes contribute to ASD.

Some of the genetic variations associated with autism show pleiotropy – they are also associated with other disorders such as

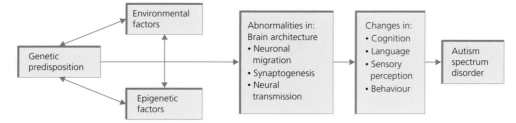

Figure 3.1 Genetic and environmental factors in the aetiology of autism.

Box 3.1 **Genetics terminology**

Penetrance The proportion of individuals with a particular variant of a disease-causing gene who express the associated phenotype. In highly penetrant conditions, a high proportion of individuals carrying the particular gene variant develop the associated disease
Copy number variation A structural phenomenon involving repetitive copies of a section of the genome. The number of repeats varies among individuals of the human population
Single nucleotide polymorphism A variation in a single nucleotide (adenine, thymine, cytosine or guanine) at a single point in the genome
Pleiotropy The phenomenon of a single gene affecting more than one phenotypic trait

---

Table 3.1 Examples of candidate genes in the aetiology of autism

Locus	Gene	Role
2q32	Neurexin 1	Encodes a membrane protein important for neurotransmission
7q36.2	Engrailed 2	Encodes a transcription factor important in the development of serotonergic and noradrenergic nuclei in the mid and hindbrain
16p11.2	Mitogen-activated protein kinase 3	Encodes a protein kinase important in intracellular cell-signalling

schizophrenia and ADHD and this probably explains why autism is associated with a number of other disorders.

Environmental factors

In addition to genetic factors, several environmental factors are thought to contribute to ASD at different stages of development (Table 3.2). However, this is often an area of controversy; for example no causal link has been found between ASD and the measles, mumps and rubella (MMR) vaccine (Box 3.2).

Another key discredited cause of ASD is a lack of parental warmth and attachment to the affected child – this was known as the 'refrigerator mother' theory. Although this theory has now been largely consigned to history, it is important to note that in some countries, such as France, it remains popular, and ASD is often attributed to poor parenting or family dysfunction.

Table 3.2 Some environmental factors thought to be involved in the aetiology of autism

Developmental stage	Examples
Prenatal	Advanced parental age
	Maternal diabetes
	Exposure to teratogens (e.g. maternal valproic acid, organophosphates)
	Infections (e.g. congenital rubella)
Perinatal	Birth asphyxia
	Prematurity
	Low birth weight
Postnatal	Hypoxia
	Autoimmune disease
	Postnatal infections
	Mercury and other environmental pollutants

Box 3.2 **Autism and the measles, mumps and rubella vaccine**

There has been much debate over the potential link between autism and the measles, mumps and rubella (MMR) vaccine. The original research paper suggesting a link between the MMR vaccine and ASD has been discredited, and a 2014 meta-analysis confirmed no relationship between ASD and MMR vaccination (OR 0.84; 95% CI 0.70–1.01) or to components of the vaccine including thiomersal (OR 1.00; 95% CI 0.77–1.31) or mercury (OR 1.00; 95% CI 0.93–1.07). However, because many people remain worried about the risks of having their child vaccinated, there is ongoing public health concern about how reduced vaccination rates could lead to an increased prevalence of preventable diseases such as measles.

Other key areas of current research on aetiology include the role of hormonal factors, and gastrointestinal and immune systems dysfunction and ASD genesis.

Conclusions

Our current understanding of the aetiology of ASD is limited. There is still much to learn about the complex genetic, epigenetic and environmental factors underlying ASD, their interplay, and how these affect brain development and function. Future research could lead to developments in ASD diagnostic tests and novel intervention targets.

Further reading

Autism Research Centre, University of Cambridge. Research Projects – Genetics and Proteomics. https://www.autismresearchcentre.com/research_projects_5. Accessed: 16 November 2018.

Boucher J. Autism Spectrum Disorder: Characteristics, Causes and Practical Issues, 2nd edn. London: Sage Publications, 2017.

Constantino J, Charman T. Diagnosis of autism spectrum disorder: reconciling the syndrome, its diverse origins, and variation in expression. Lancet Neurology 2016; 15: 279–291.

de Kluiver H, Buizer-Voskamp JE, Dolan CV, Boomsma DI. Paternal age and psychiatric disorders: a review. American Journal of Medical Genetics Part B: Neuropsychiatric Genetics 2017; 174: 202–213.

Grafodatskaya D, Chung B, Szatmari P, Weksberg R. Autism spectrum disorders and epigenetics. Journal of the American Academy of Child and Adolescent Psychiatry 2010; 49: 794–809.

Kern JK, Geier DA, Sykes LK, Boyd EH, Geier MR. The relationship between mercury and autism: a comprehensive review and discussion. Journal of Trace Elements in Medicine and Biology 2016; 37: 8–24.

Taylor LE, Swerdfeger AL, Eslick GD. Vaccines are not associated with autism: an evidence-based meta-analysis of case–control and cohort studies. Vaccine 2014; 32: 3623–3629.

Warrier V, Chee V, Smith P, Chakrabarti B, Baron-Cohen S. A comprehensive meta-analysis of common genetic variants in autism spectrum conditions. Molecular Autism 2015; 6: 49.

CHAPTER 4

The Features of Autism in Childhood

Munib Haroon

OVERVIEW

- The features suggestive of autism spectrum disorder can usually be recognised from an early age.
- The core features may always not be obvious in younger children; sometimes they may only become noticeable in adolescence, or even adulthood – when new stressors come into play or where social demands exceed a person's abilities.
- It is important to interpret possible autistic features in the context of a child's developmental age and ability.
- The presentation in females can be different from that in males and can lead to diagnostic delay.

First concerns

The symptoms, signs and areas of difficulty seen in autism are protean: there is no single feature pathognomonic of the condition.

The core features of autism (Figure 4.1) relate to the dyad of impairments (social communication/social interaction difficulties and restricted, repetitive patterns of behaviour, interests and activities) but, in addition to these, children with autism can present with many other generalised or non-specific features – especially at a younger age (e.g. speech delay).

Children also present with features resulting from co-morbid or associated conditions, such as ADHD, anxiety disorders, mood disorders, epilepsy and developmental co-ordination disorder. When these are present in a child with undiagnosed autism, and when marked, they can mask and make it difficult to pick up on the presence of autistic signs. It is therefore important for a clinician to have a high index of suspicion about related disorders when seeing the signs of one and to not put all their eggs into one 'diagnostic basket'.

Normal development

There is a broad range of normality when it comes to the development of speech and social communication and social interaction skills. It is important that clinicians are able to recognise when development is within the normal range and when it is not. Development can be delayed – meaning it is following normal pathways but happening later than expected – or it can be disordered. Both delayed and disordered development can occur together. An appreciation of what is normal (and how broad a term it is) only comes through experience of working with children of different ages and abilities. 'Typical' time periods for the development of speech, communication and socialisation skills are shown in Table 4.1.

What is normal for a child at one age can be abnormal at another age. For example, lack of single-word speech in a 2-year-old would be worrying and could indicate that the child needs to be assessed for autism whereas it would not be similarly concerning in a 9-month-old child. The very young present additional diagnostic challenges for the clinician. For example, those below 2 years can present with non-specific signs rather than features typically associated with autism; as such, it is difficult to be clear what the minimum age is for making a reliable diagnosis.

Because the features change according to age, it is helpful to consider how children with autism present in different age ranges – for example in pre-school children, school-aged children and older adolescents. There is, of course, much overlap between these groups, and the latter will also have features in common with adults (who are considered in a separate chapter).

Male and female

There can also be differences in presentation between the genders: females often have subtler difficulties with social communication and social interaction. This may be because girls with autism intrinsically have fewer difficulties in these areas to begin with, or because as they grow up they learn to 'mask' them (some describe girls with autism as being effective 'social mimics' or 'little philosophers'). There can also be qualitative differences in interests, for example young girls with autism can be very interested in animals or dolls –which can easily be passed over as not being relevant to a diagnosis. Finally, difference between the sexes, in terms of the presentation of co-morbid conditions (e.g. ADHD), can compound

---

ABC of Autism, First Edition. Munib Haroon.
© 2019 John Wiley & Sons Ltd. Published 2019 by John Wiley & Sons Ltd.

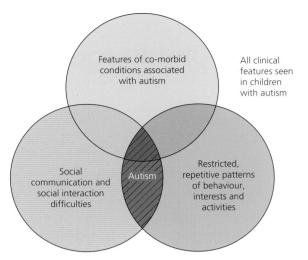

Figure 4.1 There are many clinical features that can be seen in children with autism. The core features of autism relate to those described by the dyad of impairments and include social communication and social interaction difficulties alongside restricted, repetitive patterns of behaviour, interests and activities. Autistic children will have difficulties in both areas and can also have features associated with other co-morbid conditions.

the difficulty in recognising that a girl or an adult woman need a referral for further assessment.

Signs of autism in the pre-school child

The features of autism can be noticed from a very young age, although parents are sometimes only able to say in retrospect that they noticed 'something wasn't right' from when their child was a baby. Whilst formal screening for autism in young children is not undertaken in the UK, it is important that health care professionals who work with young children are aware of the signs and features of autism so that they are able to take appropriate action when they see a child who requires further assessment.

Some of the signs and features associated with autism in the pre-school child are shown in Box 4.1.

Children in whom concerns about autism are raised may show many of these features or only a few, and, as has already been stressed, they may not be at all obvious during a short clinical appointment. As such, if there is doubt about what a parent is describing and about the need for further assessment it is important to seek further information – for example from pre-school. This can often be obtained in the

Table 4.1 Speech, communication and socialisation at different ages.

6 months	1 year	18 months	2 years	3 years	4 years
Turns towards familiar voices, and listens to voices that are not in view	Responds to own name immediately	Uses 6–20 words and understands many more	Uses 50 or more words. Can join 2 words together to form a simple sentence	Modulated speech for loudness and pitch, but will still talk to self in monologues	Completely intelligible speech
Regards and follows parental faces	Babbles with vowels and some consonants. Follows the gaze of an adult	Can request using point *and* vocalisation, and look to see if an adult has understood	Refers to self by name or 'me' Talks to self in long monologues to self. Repetitive speech	Can reference emotions and show empathy	Understands jokes and has a sense of humour
Recognises facial expressions (e.g. happy)	Plays pat a cake and can wave 'bye bye'	Can obey simple instructions – 'hold my hand'	Simple role play. Can take turns. Plays alongside other children but not with them	Imaginative play including make believe play with other children. Able to share toys	More developed imagination. Enjoys dressing up

Box 4.1 **Some of the signs and symptoms of autism in pre-school children**

- There can be a delay or absence of spoken language. The extent of this can be variable and may become clinically apparent in little time or require detailed assessment and exploration to look for alternative causes as well as autism. In older pre-school children, speech patterns which may be normal at an earlier age may persist or stand out, such as repetitive speech or echolalia.
- Children may be reported as not being able to read facial expressions or to respond appropriately to them. In a similar vein, they may appear to stare through or past people.
- Eye contact may be unusual. A child may avoid making eye contact or not mesh it in the normal way when using speech, expressions and gestures (e.g. children normally use voice and eye contact to gain a person's attention whilst they point to an object of interest).
- Aspects of socialisation may be impaired in a number of ways: showing interest in adults and other children, turn taking, initiating activities such as social play, and sharing toys or other objects of interest and enjoyment. (Girls with autism may seem more social than their boy counterparts – at least superficially.)
- Imagination can seem to be impaired, with reduced or absent pretend play.
- Unusual hand/finger or other motor mannerisms such as rocking, spinning or tip-toe walking may be noticeable.
- Changes in routine can lead to children becoming anxious or overly upset – for example, if their route to nursery changes.
- Abnormal interests. Young children may not play with toys in the normal manner – for example, they may not play imaginatively with action figures, or may only be interested in playing with particular toys (to the point that their play seems to be obsessive), or they may only be interested in parts of toys or other objects, or in lining them up rather than actually playing with them.
- Sensory interests or avoidance of certain sensory stimuli can be particularly noticeable. This includes a dislike of certain sounds (hoovers, fireworks, children crying) and/or a dislike of tactile (socks, clothes, having hair washed), gustatory and visual stimuli.

form of a report or through the use of an autism specific screening instrument. Sometimes, a longer period of clinical observation – for example by arranging to see a child for a second time can also be helpful. Some of these features lead to children being described as 'just naughty' by teachers or carers, but whilst autistic children, like all children, *can* be naughty, it is important not to accept the label of 'naughty' without attempting to scratch beneath the surface – after all, can 'naughtiness' ever really be understood and managed if separated from its underlying cause and explanation?

School-aged children

The difficulties experienced by autistic school-aged children can be markedly varied according to their age, their individual personas and the presence of any associated medical conditions (Box 4.2). As a child grows, the difficulties experienced during pre-school may persist, become more noticeable or change in character. Sometimes the difficulties become less noticeable over time and may only be prominent during times of stress or during transitions.

Older adolescents

There is a large amount of overlap between the autistic features described for younger children and those that occur in adolescents. In addition, many adolescents, especially older ones, will have features similar to those seen in adults. It is helpful to refer to the tables for school-aged children and adults (see Chapter 9).

Adolescence is marked by hormonal changes and an increasing complexity in academic work, social demands – including personal relationships – as well as the pressure of exams, and then by leaving school and the family home to start college, university or work. These stressors, which can occur together, can be effective in unmasking what have been hitherto background and unnoticed autistic features, and in triggering associated conditions such as anxiety and mood disorders.

The Boy

Sometimes sitting down to dwell
I recall a boy, a 'ne'er-do-well'
Some said he was beyond all hope:
'Has he any chance? The answers nope!'

At school he could not concentrate
White food alone went on his plate
His spidery writing crawled off the pages
And he flew into such terrible rages

He couldn't stand the slightest change
Which others wouldn't find so strange
But at other times he'd not engage
His mood could be quite hard to gauge

The slightest noise would set him off
A baby's cry, a teacher's cough.
For numbers he had a strange compulsion
His maths skills saved him from expulsion

Some called him bad, some called him naughty
Some said, 'he talks like he's nearly forty!'
So, they sent him to see us one fine day
Asking, 'will the naughtiness ever go away?'

And after much thought and pause
We finally found what was the cause
The source of all the angst and schism –
He wasn't bad: he had autism.

Box 4.2 Some of the signs and symptoms of autism in school-aged children

- Speech abnormalities These include ongoing delays in normal development which range from mild difficulties to a complete absence of speech. Other features of speech often seen include repetitive speech, echolalia; abnormalities of volume, tone, stress, or speed; abnormal use of pronouns, the use of unusual vocabulary including neologisms ('made-up' words) and advanced language. Some children are reluctant to use speech in a social setting whilst other appear over-garrulous and find it hard to stop talking about certain topics. Speech can appear overly formal, and some children are described as 'little professors'.
- Understanding can be impaired with some children having a very literal understanding of language and not understanding sarcasm or metaphors.
- Non-verbal communication, such as the use of eye contact, expression and gesture, can be impaired.
- Socialisation difficulties include problems with initiating or joining in with others at play or doing other activities. Children can have difficulties with obeying commonly understood social norms (such as invading the personal space of others or not tolerating the invasion of their personal space, or difficulty with being quiet in a library). They can become overwhelmed in groups, and can display qualitative abnormalities in how they relate to peers or adults – this can include an aversion towards such persons or being noticeably overfriendly. Girls may have a more subtle presentation and by this age have learnt to mask some of their difficulties.
- Routines can be problematic in this age group, as with younger children, although some children hide these better than others with increasing maturity. Some children's difficulties in managing with changes to their routine may not be noticed at home or at school if both environments are rigidly organised and predictable, and it is only when an unexpected change happens (a new supply teacher) or during times of transition (going abroad on holiday, changing school) that the issue is unmasked.
- Unusual interests As with younger children, an autistic child can have normal interests which are abnormally intense (collecting Star Wars figures but only Star Wars figures and nothing but Star Wars figures and only talking about these); or have somewhat unusual interests for a child of that age (an 8-year-old who is interested in *The Titanic* and knows where it was made, when it sank – down to the precise time – and how many passengers survived), or their interests may be deep but fragmented (they know 'all about' Second World War tanks but not when the war started or why or which countries were involved). In girls, a very deep, or almost 'obsessive' interest in animals or pets can easily be missed and passed over as 'something all girls are interested in' but it is the degree of interest that should be picked up on as being unusual.
- Sensory interests These can be of a similar nature to those in younger children.

Further reading

National Institute for Health and Clinical Excellence. Autism Spectrum Disorder in under 19s: recognition, referral, and diagnosis. NICE guideline CG128. London: NICE, 2011. Available from: https://www.nice.org.uk/guidance/cg128. Accessed: 16 November 2018.

Scottish Intercollegiate Guidelines Network (SIGN). SIGN 145: assessment, diagnosis and interventions for autism spectrum disorders. Edinburgh: SIGN, 2016. Available from: https://www.sign.ac.uk/assets/sign145.pdf. Accessed: 15 November 2018.

Sharma A, Cockerill H. Mary Sheridan's From Birth to Five Years. Abingdon: Routledge, 2014.

CHAPTER 5

The Assessment and Diagnosis of Autism in Children

Munib Haroon

OVERVIEW

- Deciding whether to refer a child for a detailed autism assessment is based on a number of factors including parental concerns, developmental and family history, clinical assessment and information from other professionals.

- An autism assessment involves building up a detailed patient profile based on a comprehensive history and examination as well as the use of other autism-specific tools and assessments.

- Blood tests and other investigations are not required routinely.

First contact

Children are brought to see their GP when a parent, grandparent, family acquaintance or teacher is concerned that the child might be showing signs of autism. These signs may have been present from a very young age but might not have been prominent enough to have raised concerns earlier in life. Sometimes the child may just have been perceived as being highly individual ('he's just Johnny!') or the parents may not have wanted to raise concerns because they feared being perceived as 'paranoid'.

Sometimes, however, concerns only crystallise in people's minds when a child is much older. This can happen for a number of reasons. Sometimes children are able to self-manage their difficulties through 'intellectualisation' until a 'trigger' leads to a 'tipping-point' and to the 'unmasking' of their autistic features. The trigger can be a change in their environment such as a new family relationship or a change of school or some other stressor or demand. Sometimes children are raised or educated in a highly structured, routinised environment which reduces the impact of some difficulties – such as those associated with a change in routines or circumstances. It is important to realise that concerns may not occur until later in life and that there are a number of reasons for this.

When a child is brought to see a health professional (like a GP) because of concerns around autism, it is important to be aware of the range of different features (as described in Chapter 3) and to enquire about them in a sympathetic manner. As always, obtaining an accurate history is vital but so is examining the child, and often the most informative part of this can just be taking the time to observe them in clinic. In a busy clinic setting with limited time there may not be an opportunity to do this in great detail, but even simple observations can be useful. It is also important to remember that the presence of some features does not mean a child has autism, and similarly an absence of features in a clinic (but where parents give a very clear history of autistic features) can indicate that the clinician needs more time to assess the child.

Alternatively, or in addition to more time, the use of a screening instrument can prove helpful (e.g., Childhood Autism Spectrum Test, CAST; Autism Spectrum Screening Questionnaire, ASSQ). However, the results of a screening instrument should not be the sole determining factor when deciding whether a referral to an autism assessment service is needed. A letter from a teacher or employer can also prove important in helping to decide whether a referral for an autism assessment is required.

At the initial GP consultation information should be gathered to help determine if a specialist assessment is required. Key areas that should be covered include: the nature of the problem and how it relates to the diagnostic criteria for ASD and the severity and scope of the problem (does it occur in one or many contexts?). If, on the basis of an initial or subsequent discussion, ASD is suspected, the patient should be referred for an autism assessment. This is not always an easy call to make and all the factors for or against a referral need to be considered carefully (Figure 5.1). Alternatively, an alternative diagnosis may need to be considered and an appropriate referral made.

Some children attending their GP surgery because of concerns around autism have a pre-existing diagnosis of a condition that is known to be associated with autism. These include the neurodevelopmental and mental health conditions shown in Box 5.3 as well as conditions like neurocutaneous disorders, Duchenne muscular dystrophy, epilepsy and a number of other genetic syndromes including Down's syndrome, fragile X, Rett's syndrome, Cornelia de Lange syndrome, Williams syndrome, Prader–Willi syndrome and Angelman syndrome. The presence of such conditions should 'lower the bar' for a referral.

ABC of Autism, First Edition. Munib Haroon.
© 2019 John Wiley & Sons Ltd. Published 2019 by John Wiley & Sons Ltd.

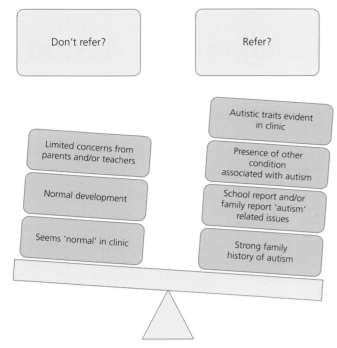

Figure 5.1 To refer or not to refer? The decision to refer for an autism assessment should be made by weighing up and exploring a number of different factors; some of these are shown in the figure. The decision to refer, however, is not always straightforward.

Specialist assessment

A specialist autism assessment is carried out by an autism team which is often based within a community paediatric or child psychiatry or Child and Adolescent Mental Health Services (CAMHS) setting, whilst in adults this is usually done in a mental health or psychiatric setting. Whether community paediatrics or CAMHS are involved depends upon local commissioning arrangements and different services can be involved for younger (community paediatrics) and for older children (CAMHS) within the same locality. Many organisations responsible for carrying out an assessment will have their own specific care pathways detailing exactly how the different processes described in this chapter are carried out.

Professionals other than an autism team can become involved in assessing a child because of another medical issue, or because a condition other than autism is suspected (e.g. hearing difficulty), or because there is insufficient evidence to warrant an assessment for autism and therefore other conditions are being investigated. Once autism is suspected an appropriate referral to the correct team via the correct referral route should take place.

Assessment by the autism team

An autism team may decide, when looking at a referral, that an autism referral is not warranted. In order to decide whether a detailed assessment should be carried out there are a number of aspects that they will consider:
- Do the reported features suggest autism?
- Are the features present in different settings?
- What is the impact that the features are having on the child and family/carer?

- What is the level of parental/carer concern?
- Is an alternative diagnosis more likely?

Where an accurate impression cannot be gauged from the referral, additional information will usually be sought by the autism team before an assessment is committed to, and this can require seeking additional information from the referrer, other health care professionals, a school or the local authority. When there is still insufficient information it may be prudent for them, in some circumstances, to meet the child/family to seek further information.

Needless back and forth between professionals has the potential to create delay, and in order to help process a referral in a time-efficient manner it is important to include relevant information on a referral the first time round. Some services have referral forms to help the referrer ensure that the relevant information has been included.

It is usual for the case to be managed by a case coordinator who will act as the point of contact for carers, patients and referrers and who tries to gather the relevant information so that an assessment can be commenced.

An autism assessment builds up a detailed profile of the patient and their environment. As such there are a number of important areas to consider (Figure 5.2). Usually, much of the information required for an assessment can be gathered by taking a history from the parents/carers and patient and carrying out a physical examination and then trying to gather additional information from professionals such as teachers.

Getting a range of views is important, because autistic features, whilst present in different settings, can be more apparent in some than in others. Additionally, it is not possible to 'spot diagnose' a child with autism, although experienced professionals will often use heuristics, consciously or subconsciously, when assessing a child and have an inkling about the outcome – and this, more often than not, may prove to be correct.

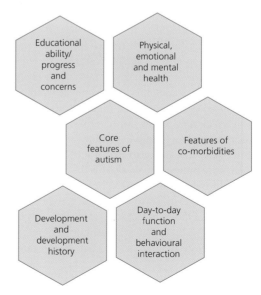

Figure 5.2 The different aspects of a patient profile that need to be built up to complete an autism assessment.

History

A detailed history that captures all the relevant information requires an appropriate setting, the right family members/carers to be present, knowing what questions to ask and enough time. It is not something that can be rushed without sacrificing important considerations, and information that is not obtained at the first appointment may have to be sought at a later date; this can lead to delay or additional and unnecessary consultation with the family. Important areas of enquiry are shown in Box 5.1.

The aim of the history in the context of an autism assessment is to help determine whether the referred child has autism or whether there are alternative explanations for their presentation, and also to enquire about possible co-morbidities and associated conditions.

The use of an autism-specific tool which relates to the ICD or DSM classifications can be used to supplement a medical history. Such tools include the Autism Diagnostic Interview – Revised (ADI-R), Developmental, Dimensional and Diagnostic Interview (3Di) and Diagnostic Interview for Social and Communication Disorders (DISCO). All such tools require training to use and can take a significant amount of time to administer. In children, the ADI-R has been shown to be reliable in aiding diagnosis whilst data on the 3Di suggests that it is comparable in performance to the ADI-R.

Examination

The examination is a vital adjunct to the history and requires experience of examining children at different ages and at different stages of development. Children with autism or other developmental or behavioural difficulties can present with certain challenges, such as severe anxiety leading to non-engagement, and these need to be anticipated and planned for. What cannot be done at the first visit may have to be rearranged for another date, but often a clear and calm explanation in pleasant surroundings with support from a parent/carer, who has brought along the child's favourite book or toy, and the support of a play therapist can work wonders. It is also important to develop the art of examining a child at a distance – by observing them and seeing how they interact with the environment and their carers.

The purpose of the examination is to tease out autistic features through observation and interaction with the child, and to help think about differential diagnoses and co-morbid conditions. It is also an opportunity to examine the child holistically and think about their general health such as growth and nutrition – which can be affected irrespective of a diagnosis of autism. Some areas to think about when examining a child are shown in Box 5.2.

Autism-specific diagnostic instruments can be used to supplement a clinical examination. These include the Autism Diagnostic Observation Schedule 2 (ADOS-2), which provides a reliable and validated way to assess a child and can be completed in approximately an hour. Autism-specific tools such as ADOS and ADI-R should be seen as supplements rather than stand-alone diagnostic instruments for an autism assessment.

Further adjuncts that can help to build up a picture of a child's strengths and difficulties and add context, and which can supplement the assessment, include obtaining information from the school or nursery and other family members and carrying out an observation in a school or home setting. Use of autism-specific tools (e.g. Gilliam Autism Rating Scale 3, GARS-3) to gather this information can be useful.

Box 5.1 **Important points of enquiry when taking a history about possible autism**

- What is the problem and in which settings does it occur? (Is it just at home, at school or in multiple settings?)
- How do the difficulties affect the child, family and peers?
- Timing: when did the issues begin, are they getting worse?
- Are there any obvious triggers for the difficulties seen?
- Which of the core features of autism are present: are there social communication and social interaction difficulties and repetitive and restricted patterns of behaviour, interests and activities?
- Are there any other associated features such as problems with sleep, seizures, feeding problems, hearing problems, self-injurious behaviours or bowel/bladder problems?
- Are there any features that suggest co-morbid conditions associated with autism such as ADHD, developmental coordination disorder, mood disorders, anxiety disorders, obsessive compulsive disorder, tics and Tourette's syndrome.
- The past medical history should include the antenatal history and enquiries should cover the use of maternal alcohol, medication, substance use as well as asking about the perinatal, birth and neonatal period. Other past medical history should be enquired about – including behavioural and emotional and mental health problems.
- Family history. As well as seeking information about any family history of autism, hearing/speech abnormalities or other developmental conditions, it is important to ask about any psychiatric history in the family such as mood and anxiety disorders, psychosis, obsessive compulsive disorder, bipolar and personality disorders.
- Developmental history. A detailed developmental history asking about delay or regression should be obtained. This can use formal developmental tool kits or be done more informally.
- Social/family history. This should include asking about the child's education and finding out about how they are managing at school, whether they have a learning disability, what supportive structures are employed and whether they have an Education, Health and Care Plan? Any current or past involvement with social services (e.g. Looked After status/safeguarding involvement) and the reasons for this are also important to ascertain. Finally, it is important to be clear on the family set-up and what changes have occurred to it in the child's lifetime and why, as well as asking about changes in housing, and family employment.

SIGN recommend that all children with autism should have a comprehensive assessment of speech/language and communication carried out, with consideration given to an assessment of their intellectual, neuropsychological and adaptive functioning. This could be carried out before the actual diagnosis has been made.

Differential diagnosis and co-morbid conditions

A full assessment should allow consideration for whether a child has autism based on the current ICD/DSM classifications (or an alternative diagnosis). Other conditions that need to be considered as alternative explanations are shown in Box 5.3. In addition, all of these differentials can occur *alongside* a diagnosis of autism along with functional problems involving feeding, sleeping, continence, constipation and visual/hearing difficulties.

Biomedical tests

In general, medical investigations should not be routinely carried out but should be considered on an individual basis, taking into account the presence of dysmorphology, neurocutaneous lesions, congenital abnormalities, intellectual disability and the likelihood of epilepsy. Where genetic testing is felt to be worthwhile, a Comparative Genomic Hybridisation (CGH) array along with DNA testing in males for fragile X is considered the first line test and yields an underlying diagnosis in 14% of individuals with ASD, when carried out routinely (95% CI = 7–22%).

Other investigations should be carried out for reasons other than to diagnose autism, such as an EEG to confirm a clinical diagnosis of epilepsy or audiology assessments to exclude a hearing impairment.

Diagnosis

A diagnosis of autism is made, or ruled out, after looking at all of the gathered information and is made in relation to the ICD or DSM classifications.

In a child with a sufficient number of chronic features involving the dyad of impairments, which are present in more than one setting and which are causing functional or other impairments and where there is no better explanation, making a diagnosis after the assessments have been completed can be relatively straightforward.

However, occasionally there can be some diagnostic uncertainty. This occurs particularly in those under 2 years, those with a developmental age of <18 months, in children where there is a lack of information about their development (e.g. looked-after or adopted children), older teenagers; those with a complex mental health disorder, a sensory disorder, cerebral palsy or other motor disorder. In children where a diagnosis is not appropriate but who nevertheless have related or other issues, referrals to alternative services should be considered. Where a diagnosis is unclear but possible, it may be relevant to consider looking at what additional assessments could help, adopting a 'wait and see' approach or considering whether a referral for a second opinion might be useful.

Irrespective of the decision, the outcome of the assessment should be communicated to the carers and, where relevant, to the patient in a clear, age-appropriate and sensitive manner. Whilst face-to-face feedback has many benefits, a written report should also be prepared, and this should be shared with the GP and with key professionals following parental consent.

Further reading

National Institute for Health and Clinical Excellence. Autism Spectrum Disorder in under 19s: recognition, referral, and diagnosis. NICE guideline CG128. London: NICE, 2011 (updated 2017). Available from: https://www.nice.org.uk/guidance/cg128. Accessed: 16 November 2018.

Scottish Intercollegiate Guidelines Network (SIGN). SIGN 145: assessment, diagnosis and interventions for autism spectrum disorders. Edinburgh: SIGN, 2016. Available from: https://www.sign.ac.uk/assets/sign145.pdf. Accessed: 15 November 2018.

CHAPTER 6

Managing Day-to-Day Issues

Munib Haroon, Monica Shaha, and Mini G. Pillay

OVERVIEW

- It is useful to have a framework for managing day-to-day behavioural difficulties.
- First defining what the problem is and then seeking to understand its triggers can be a good starting point.
- There are a number of useful strategies that parents can be taught to manage the child's behavioural difficulties.
- Behavioural strategies should be tried before medication is considered.
- Behaviourisms can be part of the core presentation of autism, related to associated co-morbid conditions, or be the result of underlying psychosocial or medical problems.

Autism cannot be cured, but many of the day-to-day issues that are problematic in an autistic child can be managed with appropriate strategies. This is a very large topic, and so this chapter provides merely a broad overview of practical techniques and approaches that professionals may find helpful to know a little bit about; whilst Chapter 16 looks at a broader range of interventions from a theoretical perspective.

A framework for addressing behaviour

There are many different approaches to managing behaviour. An approach which is easy to understand and which can be modified by parents, begins by asking what the problem is (Figure 6.1).

Useful general strategies

There are a number of useful general strategies that can be used to manage or pre-empt problem behaviours and to help with learning. These are shown in Box 6.1.

Managing social communication and social interaction difficulties

Children with autism struggle with social interaction and social communication but sometimes the problem is not due to the 'core features' of autism. Children with autism may be having problems with concentration, anxiety or too much sensory stimulation. As a result, it is always important, when seeking to manage a problem, to think about the general framework for managing behaviour and to first define what the problem is and to seek to understand why it is happening.

There are a number of areas where children may need help, and there are a number of simple strategies that can be tried (Table 6.1) in addition to some of the strategies that have been outlined already. However, the evidence base for them may not always be well established. Often the key is having a plan, persistence by parents or caregivers, keeping the goals achievable, using lots of praise and using as many visual strategies as possible.

Stereotypies

Stereotypies are movements often seen in autism, which are often confused with tics (Table 6.2). They can be disabling and lead to social stigma, impair access to education and sometimes lead to self-injury. Examples are rocking, head banging, arm flapping, waving and arm shaking. Children do not usually find these movements unpleasant or intrusive and they often reduce in frequency as the child gets older. Doing something to address them is not always necessary but might need to be considered if the behaviours are getting in the way of life, are attracting undue attention (e.g. from bullies) or are hurting someone.

Parents and professionals can help the child overcome these issues in a number of ways (Box 6.2). It is also important to think about the general behaviour management framework.

ABC of Autism, First Edition. Munib Haroon.
© 2019 John Wiley & Sons Ltd. Published 2019 by John Wiley & Sons Ltd.

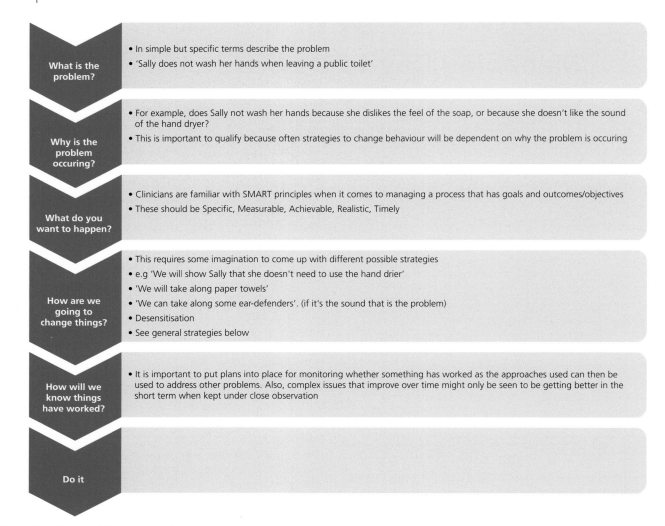

What is the problem?
- In simple but specific terms describe the problem
- 'Sally does not wash her hands when leaving a public toilet'

Why is the problem occuring?
- For example, does Sally not wash her hands because she dislikes the feel of the soap, or because she doesn't like the sound of the hand dryer?
- This is important to qualify because often strategies to change behaviour will be dependent on why the problem is occuring

What do you want to happen?
- Clinicians are familiar with SMART principles when it comes to managing a process that has goals and outcomes/objectives
- These should be Specific, Measurable, Achievable, Realistic, Timely

How are we going to change things?
- This requires some imagination to come up with different possible strategies
- e.g 'We will show Sally that she doesn't need to use the hand drier'
- 'We will take along paper towels'
- 'We can take along some ear-defenders'. (if it's the sound that is the problem)
- Desensitisation
- See general strategies below

How will we know things have worked?
- It is important to put plans into place for monitoring whether something has worked as the approaches used can then be used to address other problems. Also, complex issues that improve over time might only be seen to be getting better in the short term when kept under close observation

Do it

Figure 6.1 A framework for managing day-to-day behavioural issues.

Box 6.1 **Useful strategies for preventing and managing behaviour**

- **The 6P's: Prior Preparation Prevents Panic and Problematic Periods** Children with autism respond better to change when warned in advance of its imminent arrival. The greater the change, the more frequent the warning may need to be (and the earlier, before the event, they may need to start). Often, such warnings work well when augmented with visual strategies. For example, a visit to the dentist may require the child to be prepped a few weeks in advance (verbally) but this may need to be augmented with an online visit to the dentist's website, and also for them to walk past the surgery and – if felt necessary – drop in to the surgery to see the layout of the room and to chat to staff.
- **Visual timetables** This can be a simple chart showing the days of the week (a.m. and p.m.) with images to shows what the child will be doing on each day. They can be used at school but also at home.
- **Desensitisation** A form of graded exposure to situations that provoke fear.
- **Chaining and backwards chaining** Chaining consists of breaking down a task into small steps and teaching/showing/going through all the steps with the child and then, next time, allowing them to do the early steps for themselves. If successful, on the subsequent attempt, the child will do more of the steps in the process. Backwards chaining is much the same except that the child does the steps at the end.
- **Positive reinforcement** The use of rewards to promote good behaviour. The rewards should be for specific behaviour ('if you put the toys on the bedroom floor into the toybox in the next ten minutes') rather than vague ones ('go tidy up'). Rewards can be toys, praise, star charts, a trip or time doing an activity. Rewards should not be too far off in time from the event that is being reinforced, and it is always helpful if the reward does not 'break the bank' financially for the parents.
- **Clear rules** Having clear rules, and set boundaries, is very important for children with autism and can stop problems from beginning in the first place. Often these need to be repeated and reiterated frequently.

Table 6.1 Strategies for managing social communication and social interaction difficulties.

Difficulty	Strategy
Understanding emotions	Parental verbalisation and explanation of feelings. ('Look, daddy is smiling, that means he is happy', or, 'you're smiling, that means you're happy!') Emotion diaries Emotional thermometer Cartoons and comics. Although there are cartoons specifically to help with this, any comic or cartoon with clearly drawn and accurately rendered facial expressions can be used to teach a child about expressions and emotions
Turn taking (in games and when speaking)	Clear explanations and 'rules' Timers ('You talk for one minute and then it is daddy's turn') The Talking Hat ('I have the hat and it is my turn to build the jigsaw. When I give you the hat it will be your turn') Teaching by example ('See, daddy is building the jigsaw, he will put in two pieces and then it will be mummy's turn')
Understanding the conventions of speech	Self-talk while the child watches. 'I am going to go into the shop and look at Mr Smith and say, "hello Mr Smith, how are you today?"' Role play Social stories. A focused story specific to the child and social situation that teaches appropriate behaviour by showing a character carrying out the right actions and being praised for them. Social stories are very flexible tools and can be used in a diverse number of situations

Table 6.2 Similarities and differences between stereotypies and tics.

Stereotypies	Tics
Repetitive, ritualistic, rhythmic movement posture or vocalisation	Sudden, involuntary, rapid, non-rhythmic, non-purposeful, motor movement or vocalisation
Occur commonly (but not exclusively) in autistic spectrum disorders	Not as strongly associated with autism
No premonitory urge prior to the behaviour	Often associated with a premonitory urge, and a feeling of relief once the tic has been performed
Can appear enjoyable	Suppression can cause tension
Somewhat fixed in their pattern	Can wax and wane; the type and site can change
Worsened by tiredness, anxiety and stress	Worsened by tiredness, anxiety and stress

Obsessions, compulsions and routines

Autistic people often use routines to create a sense of predictability and security in, what is to them, an unpredictable world. Before tackling obsessions and routines, it is useful to ask the following questions:
- Does the obsession or routine impact on the child's development by restricting social or learning opportunities?

Box 6.2 **Strategies for managing stereotypies**

- Not everything can be addressed simultaneously. Making a list of behaviours hierarchically, from ones that are easy to modify to those that will be more tricky, can help form a plan of action.
- Identify when and where the stereotypies occur and the triggers for them. Are they linked to boredom, anxiety, sensory-seeking behaviour? It can be useful to try to minimise triggers. If a problem is caused by anxiety then helping the child with anxiety strategies, such as relaxation techniques or distraction, can be useful, as can providing an alternative response or behaviour that the child can engage with (e.g. by playing with a small toy).
- If the behaviour is safe to do when he/she is alone, providing the child with a private space where he/she can safely engage in the behaviours at an appropriate time can also be useful.
- Remember that some behaviours may not diminish and will have to be accepted.
- Refer to a specialist service if there is doubt about diagnosis, or if medication is being considered.

- Is the routine impractical, not only for the child but also for the family?
- Does it cause distress or discomfort to the child?
- Is it unsafe?

If the answer is 'no', there may be no need to intervene. If the answer is 'yes' to any of the above questions, the child will need support to diminish the behaviour.

If it is felt that the behaviour needs to be diminished, consider the behaviour management framework in Figure 6.1 and the following points:
- What does the child get out of it? Is it to block out sensory stimuli (e.g. noise), to seek sensation (e.g. rubbing a piece of cloth repeatedly) or to relieve anxiety? Often, it is a combination of reasons and these may all need to be addressed in turn.
- Is a change of environment needed? Perhaps the classroom is too noisy or too bright? Can strip lighting be used? Can the child have a 'safe' space at home that is suited to his/her needs?
- Increased structure and predictability. This can be helpful if the routine, obsession or compulsion has developed because of anxiety around change. In this situation, using a visual timetable for the day ahead or using egg-timers to count down to a transition (e.g. when it is time to start brushing teeth before bed), or other strategies to lessen anxiety can be helpful.
- Intervene early – the longer a routine or obsession is established, the harder it is to modify.
- Set clear, firm boundaries – for example, set a limit to the length of time the child can spend talking about the obsession or routine, set a limit to the places where he/she can carry it out.
- Rewarding desired behaviour. This can be a useful way to shape the child's behaviour in a different direction. Again, having a SMART approach (Specific, Measurable, Achievable, Realistic, Timely), aiming for modest change and being persistent can be key.

Box 6.3 **When to be concerned about a child's eating**

- If the child is accepting fewer than 20 foods
- If the child refuses all foods from one or more food groups
- If the child presents with constipation
- If the child presents with tooth decay as a result of the diet
- Weight loss or failure to thrive
- Excessive weight gain
- Behaviour suggesting deficiency of a food group or other dietary element, for example tiredness or pica (eating non-edible items), which might indicate a vitamin or mineral deficiency (e.g. iron deficiency anaemia)
- Missing school because of eating problems
- Coughing and choking while eating, or having recurrent chest infections, especially in the presence of developmental delay or physical disabilities
- Missing out on social opportunities, for example if the child and family can rarely go out because of the eating problems

Box 6.4 **Helpful mealtime strategies for children with ASD**

- Have a regular pattern and time for meals in a regular location
- Establish a calm and comfortable environment with appropriate table and seating
- Reduce unnecessary sensory distractions. Music and TV can help, but also hinder
- Sitting with others who are eating helps some, whilst others concentrate best when they are not being watched
- Work to broaden the variety of diet by initially expanding on already accepted food groups (e.g. different types of breads)
- Try to apply general strategies (Table 6.1) – for example, visual supports and positive reinforcement

Eating difficulties

In children, rigidity around foods is very common – not just for those on the autism spectrum. In general, there is no need to be too concerned if the child is eating foods from each of the main food groups and is growing well. Advice should be sought, however, if this is not happening or in the presence of other concerning features (Box 6.3). There are a number of helpful strategies that can be employed on a proactive basis to help problematic behaviour from becoming ingrained or to help with alleviation, especially before it becomes severe and professional input is required (Box 6.4).

Sleep difficulties

Sleep difficulties are very common in children with autism. The problems range from insufficient sleep, to difficulty in settling, or waking up in the middle of the night or in the early hours. This can lead to tiredness and impact upon learning and behaviour in general. It can also have a very significant effect upon parents and siblings.

Addressing sleep issues should be done with an eye on the framework for managing behaviour. Understanding any possible underly-

Box 6.5 **Factors that affect sleep in a child with autism**

- Anxiety
- Repetitive thoughts
- Sensory difficulties
- Hyperactivity
- Lack of routine
- Daytime sleep
- Caffeine
- Inappropriate environment
- Medical causes (obstructive sleep apnoea, asthma)

Box 6.6 **Case vignette: Adnan**

Adnan, aged 9, was referred to the paediatrician because he was awake until midnight and then waking up at 6 a.m. The doctor took a careful history and suggested that the family try a couple of measures and see if that helped. On the basis of the doctor's advice, Adnan's parents added a blackout blind to his bedroom and restricted use of his iPad from 8 p.m. onwards. In addition, Adnan had a last cup of tea at 4 p.m. – all this helped his sleep. When he returned to the paediatrician, Adnan also admitted that he was worrying about being bullied, and when this was addressed Adnan was asleep by 9 p.m. and his parents felt he was a lot less tired and happier in general.

ing triggers or factors (Box 6.5) for the sleep difficulty is very important because if they are ignored then improving things can prove difficult.

In addressing sleep difficulties, the concept of sleep hygiene is very important and whilst it may not solve the problem in every case, it should form a baseline for management before reaching for the prescription pad (Box 6.6).

Often, however, despite all the attention directed towards behavioural strategies, a medical approach is required. There is evidence that melatonin is effective in reducing sleep problems in children with autism. However, there are several important caveats to be borne in mind:
- Melatonin should not be used until behavioural interventions have been tried.
- Melatonin should be prescribed by a professional with the requisite expertise.
- Prescribing should be done in conjunction with the *BNF for Children* and appropriate national guidance.
- Medication should be reviewed regularly with regard to efficacy and side effects.
- Little is known about the long-term side effects and therefore appropriate caution should be used and parents informed about possible side effects and long-term concerns.

Sensory difficulties

Children with autism can have a wide range of sensory interests and difficulties which are now recognised as a part of the core presentation of autism. These can affect all five senses: hearing, vision, touch, taste and smell. Whilst not every sensory issue is a difficulty, often the sensory aspects of autism can be significantly disabling and can impact upon communication and interaction, education, sleep and other day-to-day activities. Many people are familiar with hypersensitivity in autism, but hyposensitivity can also be an area of difficulty.

There are a number of strategies that can be tried by carers to help support children with these sorts of difficulties (Box 6.7). In addition, there are a number of sensory-based training programmes and therapies; however, the evidence to support their efficacy is at this point limited. Nevertheless, in addition to day-to-day strategies, children may benefit from seeing an occupational therapist to advise their families on how to modify their environment and daily activities.

It is important to appreciate that sensory overstimulation can be exhausting for children and young people, and often having a place of 'refuge' at home and in school can be very important. In addition, it is important that after being in an overstimulating environment there is time to recharge in a tranquil setting.

Anticipation and being forewarned of adverse sensory stimuli can also help, as children and young people can mentally prepare for an event much better if they know it is coming.

Autism and the internet

Many children (and adults) with autism seem to be particularly drawn towards gaming, the internet and social media. This can lead to excessive amounts of time being spent in front of a computer, sometimes on topics of interest that then become unhealthy or inappropriate obsessions, and can lead to less time for face-to-face friendships, relationships and the opportunity to enhance socialisation skills; it can also take time away from doing homework and affect sleep. Clear rules around when computers and tablets can be used may thus need to be implemented – ideally at the outset of their use, before a problem becomes ingrained.

But the internet also has many benefits for education, networking, socialisation and entertainment – for everyone – and it can allow children with autism to interact widely with other people from a 'safe space' at home and to develop friendships with like-minded individuals or those who share a common interest. However, the 'safe space' does connect directly to a wider world which alongside its positive aspects also poses threats to everyone, including those with autism – who can be especially vulnerable to bullies and other predators. A preventative approach is preferable to dealing with a problem once it has occurred, and so education and explanation can be important in helping a young person to understand and deal with the threats posed. Using appropriate safety, security and privacy internet settings is important and in some circumstances supervised use or completely restricting access to the internet can be required. It is also important for children and young people with autism to know when to turn for help and who they can turn to. It is also important for them, as well as carers, to realise that sometimes problems can only be addressed by involving other agencies: this includes schools, social workers and the police.

Rarely (but in well-publicised cases), young people (or adults) with autism have also landed on the wrong side of the law through 'hacking' and once again prevention is better than 'cure'.

It is important to end by saying that not only is computing and information technology something that can be helpful for those with autism, but it exists in the shape it does thanks in no small part to those with autism.

Box 6.7 **Strategies to help children with sensory difficulties**

- **Sound** Children can find certain sounds unpleasant or overstimulating. Sometimes it is possible to avoid these sounds (e.g. fireworks); however, this is not always possible. For some sounds, a desensitisation approach can occasionally work to reduce apprehension (e.g. the handdriers in public toilets) whilst for others it may be necessary to use ear plugs or defenders or to rely on earphones or music. Certain environments are busier and hence noisier at certain times of the day. For example, it may be better to catch a bus into town first thing on a Saturday morning, rather than waiting until the afternoon, especially if there is a football match on and there will be large crowds in town.
- **Vision** Sunglasses can be useful outdoors as can a hat with a broad brim. Indoors, appropriate lighting may need to be investigated. Sometimes the overstimulation comes not from light but from a busy environment, such as a very crowded classroom with items hanging from walls and ceilings. This may need to be modified to take the needs of children with autism into account. Despite these modifications, a classroom or other setting can at times become 'too much' and some sort of quiet space can help to settle the child or young person.
- **Touch** Children and young people can have difficulty with having their hair cut, nails clipped and with the texture of certain clothes or their component parts (seams, zips and studs). It is important to recognise and accept this as a problem and to try to see what alternatives there are rather than insist that a child must manage as they are. Desensitisation and graded exposure can help in some areas as can providing explanations, warnings or using rewards for tolerating certain scenarios ('because you were brave when we cut your nails'). It is important to experiment and not to think that there is no solution to the difficulty. Tactile issues can also be important when it comes to toileting. Children may not like the feel of a particular type of toilet seat, the feel of a dirty nappy or how passing a stool feels. Alternatively, they can be intensely interested in the feel of faecal matter and this can lead to them smearing stool. In addressing such issues it is important to begin with the most important questions: what is the problem, and why is it happening? Is it a sensory issue, or it caused by something else?
- **Taste** Difficulties with taste can lead to children having a restricted diet, which can sometimes affect growth, or which can cause stress for families even if there is no other medical problem. A useful approach is to introduce new tastes one at a time, using small portions and providing plenty of warning that a new food is to be tried. Giving praise and rewards can be helpful.
- **Smell** It is possible to avoid certain smells, but not all of them. Sometimes having something to carry around to act as a distraction (a toy) can be useful as can having an alternative scent in a spray bottle which can be used in a discrete manner.

Further reading

Association of UK Dieticians. Available from: https://www.bda.uk.com/foodfacts/autism. Accessed: 19 November 2018.

National Autistic Society. Eating. Available from: www.autism.org.uk/about/health/eating.aspx. Accessed: 19 November 2018.

National Autistic Society. Obsessions, repetitive behaviour and routines. Available from: www.autism.org.uk/about/behaviour/obsessions-repetitive-routines.aspx#. Accessed: 22 November 2018.

National Autistic Society. Staying safe online. Available from: https://www.autism.org.uk/staying-safe-online. Accessed: 19 November 2018.

Silberman S. Neurotribes. London: Allen and Unwin, 2015.

Williams C, Wright B. How to Live with Autism and Asperger's Syndrome. London: Jessica Kingsley, 2004.

CHAPTER 7

Mental Health in Children With Autism

Monica Shaha and Mini G. Pillay

OVERVIEW

- Coexisting mental health problems including anxiety, ADHD and depression are common in children with a diagnosis of ASD.

- When working with children who have autism, a clinician should have a low threshold for suspecting the presence of other co-morbid diagnoses.

- Medication is not always the first line treatment for mental health co-morbidity and does not treat the underlying condition.

- The main advice with medication use for children is to 'start low, go slow'.

Autism is a complex disability that by definition presents with social communication and social interaction difficulties. These difficulties pose a number of challenges to the recognition, evaluation and treatment of mental health problems especially in children where the difficulties in expressing thoughts, feelings and emotions can be compounded by a young age.

Epidemiology

Estimates vary, but according to one study, about 70% of children with autism develop mental health conditions, with an anxiety disorder or phobia occurring in about 40% and ADHD in about 30%. This compares to an overall prevalence rate of around 10% in other children. A more recent study carried out by the National Autistic Society (You Need to Know, 2010) looked at the most commonly reported mental health problems and found that anxiety was the most frequent difficulty (Table 7.1).

Assessment – general principles

When to suspect psychiatric co-morbidity

Given the high incidence of associated co-morbidities in autism, it is important to have a low threshold for suspecting that one or more conditions may be present. In the primary care setting remembering this and referring the child on for further detailed assessment is

therefore a crucial first step, and so it is important to be aware of the features that suggest that something else in addition to autism is present. Some of these general indicators are outlined in Box 7.1.

Diagnostic overshadowing

Once a diagnosis is made of a major condition there is a tendency to attribute all other problems to that diagnosis, thereby leaving other coexisting conditions undiagnosed.

As an example, social withdrawal resulting from a developing depressive illness or anxiety caused by an anxiety disorder may be wrongly attributed as being related to the child or young person's autism. This can be further compounded because different services may be involved (sometimes at the same time) in diagnosing and managing autism and in diagnosing and managing mental health difficulties (e.g community paediatrics and CAMHS).

This process can also work in the other direction, with conditions such as ADHD and anxiety overshadowing the underlying or associated diagnosis of autism.

Specific conditions

Depression and ASD

Depression, which is typically characterised with low mood, can be hard to recognise in autistic children; however, it is a common presentation that should not be allowed to go unrecognised because of the impact it can have upon many aspects of life. This includes the enjoyment of day-to-day activities, sleep, friendships and educational attainment. Individuals with autism can find it difficult to identify, name and communicate to others the feelings of sadness, guilt or shame that are typically associated with a depressive illness. Consequently, cases are often reported by a carer or a professional involved with the child or young person.

Presenting features include increased irritability, altered facial expression, altered behavioural patterns and loss of interest in usual activities. Children and young people with autism can have restricted diets, as well as sleep disturbances that are related to their autism. However, any change in the usual pattern of appetite and/or sleep is significant when screening for possible depression.

ABC of Autism, First Edition. Munib Haroon.
© 2019 John Wiley & Sons Ltd. Published 2019 by John Wiley & Sons Ltd.

Table 7.1 The most commonly reported mental health problems in autistic children.

Issue	Frequency of reporting (%)
Anxiety	85
Behavioural issues: defiance, non-compliance	62
Depression	36
Self-harm and self-injury	33
Suicidal thoughts	27
Obsessive compulsive disorder	21

Box 7.1 Signs that should lead a person to suspect that a child with autism may have a psychiatric co-morbidity

- When the child presents with (mental health) signs and symptoms outside of the core features of autism
- A deterioration in the core features of autism
- An abrupt change from a child's baseline behaviour
- A severe and incapacitating problematic behaviour (e.g. one that significantly interferes with social functioning)
- When the child does not respond as expected to usual interventions

---

Box 7.2 Triggers for anxiety

- Change, such as major events like starting or changing school or minor ones like a change in teacher. Routine is essential for autistic children as it enables their world to be structured and predictable
- Sensory over-stimulation, such as in a dining room at lunchtime, where there may be a variety of smells, loud chatter and laughter, chairs scraping and lots of people moving about. A classroom can also be full of distracting sensory elements, especially when full of children
- Anxiety can occur during unstructured sessions (e.g. playtime)
- Difficulty understanding emotions – children with autism not only struggle to understand their own emotions, but can also experience them in a different way from others, for example being excited about a party which may evolve into anxiety then present as challenging behaviour

---

Because many of these features may be subtle in their presentation or assumed to be part of the autism condition, they may go unrecognised; a clinician should always remember to ask about such features and suspect depression when they are present.

Anxiety and ASD

In the clinical setting, anxiety-related concerns are among the most common presenting problems for school-aged children and adolescents with ASD. There can be a number of triggers and these are shown in Box 7.2.

ADHD and ASD

ADHD is defined by difficulties in attention, hyperactivity and impulsivity. People with ADHD show a persistent pattern of inattention and/or hyperactivity–impulsivity that interferes with functioning or development. Additional criteria that must be met when making a diagnosis of ADHD, according to DSM-5, include the presence of several key symptoms for more than 6 months in multiple settings. A diagnosis should take a young person's developmental progress, and the presence of symptoms before the age of 12 years, into account. Like autism, 'pure' ADHD can present with sensory difficulties and socialisation difficulties – although the latter result from the core features of inattention, hyperactivity and impulsivity rather than difficulties with social understanding.

The symptoms of ADHD can significantly delay the recognition of autism in children. Symptoms of inattention and hyperactivity leading to disruptive behaviour can become obvious before the difficulties with social communication and repetitive behaviours associated with autism. As a result, ADHD symptoms can overshadow the core symptoms of autism, making the diagnosis particularly challenging to recognise in these children and calling for a high degree of vigilance.

Autism and OCD

The essential features of obsessive compulsive disorder (OCD) are the presence of recurrent obsessional thoughts or compulsive acts. These can occur in children with and without autism. The features of OCD and the restricted and repetitive patterns of behaviour, interests and activities inherent to autism can be similar enough to make distinguishing between the two conditions extremely difficult, leading to erroneous overdiagnosis of OCD in people with autism.

In both cases there can appear to be a fixation on routine, ritualised patterns of verbal and non-verbal behaviour, resistance to change and highly restrictive interests. However, the features of autism are usually present from early in life as opposed to OCD where symptoms generally have a time of onset well beyond infancy. Unlike autism, where repetitive activities can be pleasurable and provide a sense of control, the obsessions and compulsions of OCD are perceived as intrusive or unpleasant, and patients will often try to resist them or develop coping strategies to manage them.

Tics in autism

Tics can occur in autism and are involuntary, rapid, non-rhythmic, non-purposeful, motor movements or vocalisations of sudden onset. Table 7.2 shows the different forms that tics may take. By appearance they can be very prominent and hard to repress. They can also be difficult to distinguish clinically from other types of repetitive behaviours.

Tourette's syndrome is a condition that can be seen alongside autism, and which is characterised by the occurrence of multiple tics – both motor and vocal – which are chronic (long-term, lasting more than a year since the first onset).

Advice on management

There are a number of helpful strategies for managing tics:
- Not calling attention to the tics
- Avoiding stress-filled situations which can exacerbate tics
- Getting enough sleep
- Giving in to the urge. Holding back a tic can sometimes lead to a flare later on, sometimes at an inconvenient moment.

Table 7.2 The different forms of tics.

	Motor tics	Vocal tics
Simple	Eye blinking Eye rolling Grimacing Shoulder shrugging Limb and head jerking Abdominal tensing	Whistling Throat clearing Sniffing Coughing Tongue clicking Grunting Animal sounds
Complex	Jumping Twirling Touching objects and other people Obscene movements or gestures (copropraxia) Repeating other people's gestures (echopraxia)	Uttering words or phrases out of context Saying socially unacceptable words (coprolalia) Repeating a sound, word or phrase (echolalia)

Medication in managing tics and Tourette's

The symptoms of Tourette's syndrome can be helped by medication even if the underlying cause is not addressed. The use of medicines in children comes with the caveat that their use should be judicious and under the supervision of secondary care (child psychiatrists or paediatricians with a special interest). The general rule where medicine is used is to 'start low, go slow'. The newer generation antipsychotics are typically tried first (e.g. risperidone). Close monitoring for side effects plus careful pre-treatment screening is essential in this age group, and is generally undertaken by secondary care clinicians.

Interventions

There are a number of interventions that can be used (Box 7.3). Whilst they are similar to the interventions used in children and adolescents without ASD, there are some key differences when applied in the autistic setting. For example, some interventions can take longer to be effective; therapeutic rapport can take longer to develop, flexibility around appointments times needs to be considered. It is important to also consider the venues where interventions are used.

Primary care and referring to CAMHS

The GP has a number of key roles in relation to a child or young person with autism and possible co-morbidity.

- **First port of call** The GP may be the first health care professional to see a child with a mental health issue and should therefore know when to suspect there is a problem and how to access appropriate help. They can also help with signposting to support services (e.g. local autism groups from the Contact a Family directory). Research has shown that with the right support, the impact of autism and other associated difficulties on a family can be reduced.
- **Keeping an open dialogue with the child's school** Schools are often a font of knowledge about a child and the GP can serve as a vital conduit, especially early on, which can help with making a prompt diagnosis.
- **Crisis management** Families can often present suddenly when a child deteriorates for no apparent reason. The GP will most likely be their first port of call. Taking a careful history of the situation is important – remembering the areas mentioned in 'Assessment' - and not forgetting that children with autism can develop appendicitis just like anyone else – but remembering that this could occur with a sudden deterioration in behaviour, which is not psychiatric in origin.
- **A long-term presence** Children with autism and mental health conditions may need to be transitioned from CAMHS to adult mental health. In this situation, the GP may be the

---

Box 7.3 **Interventions for ASD-related psychiatric co-morbidities**

Psychosocial/non-therapeutic/non-pharmacological interventions
Useful for different co-morbid presentations
These can take the form of parent support groups, visual timetables, social stories, pictures/postcards, books ('200 tips and strategies'), dietary changes, exercise and the use of hobbies

Cognitive behavioural therapy
Useful for anxiety, OCD and depression
Autistic children struggle with understanding other points of view, so the typical application of CBT techniques may be less effective. The therapist may need to increase the use of visual aids, increase the emphasis on practical coping strategies and reduce the use of abstract language

Pharmacological interventions
Initiation of psychotropic medication in under-18s should only be carried out under the guidance of a child and adolescent psychiatrist or paediatrician. Prescribing should be carried out with reference to the *BNF/Children's BNF* and by using appropriate guidance (NICE). A helpful rule of thumb is to start low and increase slowly, and monitor carefully for side effects

Specific medications and indications
Selective serotonin reuptake inhibitors (SSRIs; used in anxiety/OCD/depression)
Antipsychotics (e.g. risperidone; used in extreme agitation, psychosis, Tourette's syndrome)
ADHD medication (e.g. methylphenidate)
Melatonin – for sleep initiation difficulties

Box 7.4 **When to strongly consider a referral to CAMHS**

- Significant risk to self (e.g. suicidal risk or significant self-harm)
- Risk of harm to others
- Challenging behaviour impacting on school/family life/social functioning
- Other symptoms impacting on school/family life/social functioning

only professional who has remained throughout the young person's 'health journey'. This can be reassuring for both the child and the family and the importance of this long-term patient-specific expertise cannot be underestimated.

It is not appropriate to refer every child with autism to CAMHS for further assessment and local or regional protocols should always be followed. Ideally, these will be linked to evidence-based national-level guidance such as that issued by NICE. However, there are some 'broad-brush' situations for when a referral to CAMHS should be strongly considered (Box 7.4).

If at all in doubt it is recommended that GPs speak either with their locality CAMHS or community paediatricians for further advice.

Further reading

Belardinelli C, Raza M, Taneli T. Comorbid behavioural problems and psychiatric disorders in autism spectrum disorders. Journal of Childhood and Developmental Disorders 2016; 2: 1–9.

Hirvikoski T, Mittendorfer-Rutz E, Boman M, Larsson H, Lichtenstein P, Bölte S. Premature mortality in autism spectrum disorder. British Journal of Psychiatry 2016; 208: 232–238.

Leitner Y. The co-occurrence of autism and attention deficit hyperactivity disorder in children – what do we know? Frontiers in Human Neuroscience 2014; 8: 268.

National Autistic Society (NAS). You need to know. London: NAS, 2010. Available from: www.autism.org.uk/get-involved/campaign/successes/you-need-to-know.aspx. Accessed 19 November 2018.

National Autistic Society (NAS). Understanding anxiety at school. London: NAS, 2017. Available from: www.autism.org.uk/professionals/teachers/classroom/understanding-anxiety.aspx. Accessed: 19 November 2018.

Schendel DE, Overgaard M, Christensen J, et al. Association of psychiatric and neurological comorbidity with mortality among persons with Autism Spectrum Disorder in a Danish population. JAMA Paediatrics 2016; 170: 243–250.

Simonoff E, Pickles A, Charman T, Chandler S, Loucas T, Baird G. Psychiatric disorders in children with autism spectrum disorders: prevalence, momorbidity, and associated factors in a population derived sample. Journal of the American Academy of Child and Adolescent Psychiatry 2008; 47: 921–929.

White SW, Oswald D, Ollendick T, Scahill L. Anxiety in children and adolescents with autism spectrum disorders. Clinical Psychology Review 2009; 29: 216–229. doi:10.1016/j.cpr.2009.01.003.

CHAPTER 8

School and Autism

Munib Haroon

OVERVIEW

- The core features of autism can lead to difficulties at school, but problems may also arise because of anxiety, low mood, poor concentration, and because of learning and physical disability.

- Problematic behaviour at school is not simply a case of someone being 'naughty'. When it occurs, the underlying triggers should be sought.

- Schools have a range of professionals that they can approach for additional advice and support.

- There are a range of measures – both small and large scale – which can help to support an individual at school. Support should be planned, introduced incrementally and monitored.

- Whilst schools operate on the basis of 'inclusion' and 'normalisation', some individuals require a special school setting or alternative arrangements.

Note: because the structures that underpin school provision vary from one country to another (even within the UK, such as between England and Scotland) this chapter focuses on general principles.

Challenges at school

Education is of central importance in every person's life. But school is not just about the academic aspects – there are also organisational and social skills to develop, friendships to make and foster, and the skill of team working to be learnt through group work and sports. Many, or all, of these areas can prove challenging for children – autistic and neurotypical alike. Sometimes, the challenge posed by school can begin even before the child reaches the classroom – whether it be whilst dealing with other peers on a school bus or whilst lining up outside the school entrance to go inside.

It is not just the core traits of autism – social communication and social interaction difficulties allied to restricted, repetitive patterns of behaviours, interest and activities — which can cause problems at school for some children. There are the challenges posed by anxiety, poor concentration, low mood, learning and physical disability (Figure 8.1).

There are many aspects of school life that can prove problematic for a child with autism (Box 8.1). For each individual it is important to try to pinpoint the issue so that it can be addressed in an appropriate manner. One of the most important things to do first is to accept that any undesirable behaviour is often not because the child is being 'naughty'. Then, it is a case of finding the underlying trigger for the behaviour, because if the response from the child is to be changed – from an 'undesirable' to a 'desirable' one – and the child supported in dealing with the behaviour, the trigger needs to be identified. Sometimes the underlying cause is obvious, but sometimes it requires a period of careful observation and for a behaviour log to be kept. It can be very helpful to ask the child and his/her parents what they think the trigger might be. Schools are generally proficient at addressing and dealing with these day-to-day issues.

Who can help?

Whilst the exact structures for providing support vary from one country to another, the overarching principles of support are similar. In England, in a mainstream school, a named member of staff – the Special Educational Needs Coordinator (SENCO) – is responsible for overseeing the provision of special educational needs. However, where additional help or advice is required by a school there are a number of professionals that schools can turn to (Box 8.2).

It is important in the context of diagnostic overshadowing, that all 'difficult' behaviour is not attributed solely to the child's autism, as it could be caused by a known or hitherto undiagnosed co-morbid condition such as ADHD, an anxiety disorder or some other unrelated medical condition or issue (e.g. tonsillitis or an ear infection). Alternatively, problems could be entirely unrelated to a medical issue of any sort (e.g. bullying or parental separation.)

ABC of Autism, First Edition. Munib Haroon.
© 2019 John Wiley & Sons Ltd. Published 2019 by John Wiley & Sons Ltd.

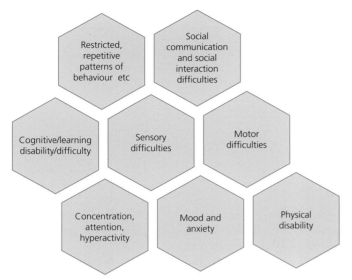

Figure 8.1 The different sorts of difficulties and problems children with autism can experience.

When a problematic behaviour is identified

When difficulties arise, the question, 'why is this happening?' should be asked. This allows for plans to be made and put into place and for progress to be monitored. Making changes to how a child is supported or taught cannot be done overnight and so it is important for teachers and parents to ask things like:

> Box 8.2 **Professionals who can provide advice to schools about a child with autism**
>
> - Special education needs teachers
> - Educational psychologists
> - Paediatricians
> - Occupational therapists/physiotherapists, speech and language therapists
> - School nurses
> - Child and adolescent psychiatrists (CAMHS)
> - Support groups and charities

> Box 8.1 **Aspects of school life that be challenging for someone with autism**
>
> - **Getting up in the morning** This can be an area of difficulty for many reasons. Many children with autism have a disrupted pattern of sleep which can lead to tiredness and poor concentration and so affect learning attainment and be associated with behavioural difficulties.
> - **Travelling to school** Some children with autism have a very set routine in how they get to school, whether it be the precise time they need to catch the bus or the route their parents take to get there. A small disruption in this can lead to a perceived over-reaction with a resulting pattern of behaviour that can last hours if not longer. Sometimes the journey on a bus with all the attendant crowding and noise, or the levels or type of social interaction taking place, can pose problems.
> - **Peer interactions at work and play** Even subtle social communication and social interaction difficulties can lead to problems with understanding other's sense of humour, sarcasm and literal interpretations of what people say. Sometimes this can lead to children with autism being 'picked on' or bullied, or to them perceiving that they are being maligned when this is not the case. Bullying can be a very significant issue and can transition onto online and social media – an arena that people with autism are often drawn towards.
> - **Lining up** Some children with autism must line up first (or in some other order); if this cannot happen and is not managed it can lead to anxiety.
> - **Carpet time** Many children with autism do not have difficulty with sitting down on a classroom carpet during an activity. For others, the close proximity to other children, the feel of the carpet or the sense that they may get dirty can lead to anxiety and other behavioural manifestations which are deemed to be disruptive.
> - **Group work** Many, if not most, children with autism prefer working alone or in very small groups to working in a group of several peers. This may be because of social communication and social interaction difficulties, although there could be sensory or other issues at play also.
> - **Transitions** Moving from one sort of activity to the next, or from one environment to the next, can be challenging for a child with autism. These can be small changes, not just large ones, and often time spent 'prepping' the child can pay dividends.
> - **Sport** Children with autism can find some sports difficult because of associated motor coordination difficulties, or because of sensory elements – such as the cold, or not wanting to get muddy – intruding upon their ability to immerse themselves in the task at hand.
> - **Individual work** This can also be an area of difficulty if the child has problems concentrating because of anxiety or inattentiveness, or because the task exceeds their cognitive ability or because of sensory overload.
> - **Exams** Children with autism can have difficulty with exams for many reasons. Concentration difficulties can hamper revision and exam performance, and raised anxiety can have a similar effect.
> - **Break time** Some of the reasons that this can be difficult include: socialisation difficulties, the unpredictable nature of the setting or because of sensory difficulties.
> - **Start/end of term** This can be a significant change in a child's routine especially with lots of different activities taking place – school trips and sports days. In a similar way a change of school can be a time of difficulty.

'Why is this happening?'

'What do we actually want to happen?'

'How are we going to change things?'

'How are we going to measure/monitor change?'

'What will we do if we don't see the change we want to see?'

There are many strategies and measures that can then be put into place to support a child with autism (Box 8.3). Some of these can be put into place more easily than others; others require the allocation of specific funds and resources to procure equipment, training or staff. It is often a case of trying things strategically, consistently and then escalating the amount of support if the child requires it. Sometimes, providing the requisite level of support needs to be done through a statutory or legal framework (Box 8.4).

Inclusivity, normalisation and setting

Thanks to the neurodiversity movement, schools nowadays operate on the basis of 'inclusivity' and 'normalisation'. These state that people with disabilities or disorders should be able to lead lives as similar as possible to those without such difficulties and that the diversity they bring to society should be welcomed and supported.

In education this translates into young people with autism being treated on an equal footing to those without autism, and for reasonable adjustments to be made where this is possible. Sometimes, however, the mainstream setting is not appropriate for a child and education needs to be provided in an alternate venue (Figure 8.2).

Box 8.3 **There are a number of supportive measures and strategies that a child with autism can find helpful**

- **Visual timetables** Can help to provide the child with a sense of order and routine. These should be appropriate to the child's age and easily accessible and up to date.
- **Fiddle toys** Can help a fidgety or sensory seeking child to focus their attention.
- **Timers** Can help to focus the child's attention for a short duration of time.
- **Appropriate seating** Making sure that the child has appropriate seating is very important. A child can benefit from being able to sit in the same seat at all times (routine). The seat should be appropriate for any physical needs and if closer to the teacher and away from distracting elements all the better.
- **Time out cards/quiet areas** Children with sensory overload or with inattention can benefit greatly from being able to leave the classroom or remove themselves to a quieter area away from other distractions.
- **1:1 support** A teaching assistant can help to focus attention and provide a closer level of supervision at school. A student can also have a scribe to help with writing for set periods, such as during exams.
- **Computers** Children with autism who also have fine motor control difficulties can find typing their work easier than handwriting. They may also be more receptive to computer-based learning.
- **Overall classroom layout** Classroom design can be improved overall so that there is less sensory overload.
- **Transport** Some children may be entitled to free transport through the council or local authority.

Box 8.4 **Case vignette: Craig**

Shortly after starting school in Birmingham, Craig was noted to be a solitary young boy who had difficulties with group play, noisy environments and listening to verbal instructions. He found it particularly difficult when there was a change in routine or a change from one activity to the next, especially if this was sudden or unexpected.

After speaking to Craig's parents, who had noted similar issues at home, the class teacher arranged a meeting with the school's Special Educational Needs Coordinator who outlined what they needed to help support Craig at school and suggested that the parents visited their GP to seek an assessment from a paediatrician. Whilst waiting for the assessment, the school put in place a range of supportive measures including the use of a visual timetable, support with play and communication, and ensured that Craig was warned of any changes to his routine. All of this was documented on his Individual Education Plan (IEP).

Over the next few terms, despite increasing levels of support, Craig experienced greater levels of difficulty, and so the SENCO spoke to his parents about applying to the local authority for an Education Health and Care Plan (EHCP). This would help to formally document Craig's educational, health and social care needs and requirements as well stating the long-term goals for him; it would also help the school to apply for additional support, allow for consistency when moving from one school to the next and allow Craig to attend a special school should this become necessary.

Although undiagnosed, the local authority decided that because the school was doing everything it could but Craig was not making progress, an EHCP would be appropriate. They decided to complete an assessment which incorporated information from the family, the school, his paediatrician and an educational psychologist. After consultation, the EHCP was completed in 20 weeks.

Towards the end of the school year Craig was assessed and given a diagnosis of autism. It was decided that a special school would be a more appropriate environment for him. His parents visited two special schools and chose the one closest to home, and after a difficult transition, Craig settled well into his new class the following September.

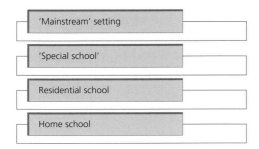

Figure 8.2 Whilst most children with autism are educated within the mainstream setting, others will need to be educated in different environments.

There is no hard and fast rule for what setting works best for a particular type of child. Each child should be assessed as an individual, taking their needs into account, as well as keeping an eye on the needs and preferences of the family.

Summary

Schools can be challenging environments for many children, but especially those who have autism. Problems should be approached by not labelling the child as naughty, and thinking about whether the behaviour is a manifestation of autism or some other underlying problem. Difficulties should be addressed strategically and systematically and the amount of support required escalated according to needs. Sometimes a statutory assessment is required and consideration given to whether a mainstream setting is the best place for the child.

Further reading

Boucher J. Autism Spectrum Disorder: Characteristics, Causes and Practical Issues, 2nd edn. London: Sage Publications, 2017.

National Autistic Society. www.autism.org.uk.

CHAPTER 9

Symptoms and Signs in Adult Autism

Alison Stansfield

OVERVIEW

- Autism in adulthood can appear very different from autism in childhood.
- The symptoms in adulthood are essentially the same as in childhood, but can be masked by maturation and intellectual ability, which enables compensatory learning and adaptation.

What does autism look like in adulthood?

To some extent this topic has already been covered in Chapter 4 but it warrants brief repetition here as autism can appear very different in adulthood. This can lead to lack of recognition and understanding and therefore a delay in assessment and subsequent diagnosis.

Autism is a syndrome consisting of behavioural symptoms, some which are typified by a lack of 'social instinct' (i.e. knowing instinctively what to do or how to behave in a social situation). Adults who present to services may have managed to negotiate life reasonably successfully, by relying on an intellectualised approach to their difficulties (observing and mimicking what others do) and can present in a variety of guises. The caricature that people with autism are train-spotters, computer technicians and engineers is far from the truth. They are just as likely to be hairdressers, physiotherapists, lecturers and doctors. The general public's perception of autism can be faulty. Autistic adults who do not have an obviously visible disability can experience intolerance when they struggle with unexpected social situations. It is to be hoped that the recent widespread media portrayal of autism will help correct this perception.

Symptoms of autism in adulthood – what to look out for

The lack of 'social instinct' seen in autism can be manifested as awkward or unusual social interaction styles (Box 9.1). If the presentation is suggestive of adult autism, especially in someone with normal or high intellect, then consider other general issues from the history or observations (Box 9.2). Although autism is characterised by a lack of 'social instinct', adults with autism, particularly women, have often become adept at watching what others do in certain situations and mimicking them (Box 9.3).

Mimicry can give the impression of the adult having instinctive social skills. Adults may appear to have natural use of non-verbal communication skills but actually may be imitating (almost immediately) the gestures and behaviour of the adult they are with. Standard social conversation often begins with 'rote language' (e.g. 'how was your journey', 'how are you doing?') which can give the false impression of natural social reciprocity and genuine interest, but difficulties arise when the topic changes to subjects relating to feelings or the interests of others and then the autistic adult becomes unable to respond and often feels excluded.

In contrast, many autistic adults, even with high intellect, do not understand the behaviour of others without autism (sometimes described by those with autism as 'neurotypicals'), so for example may arrive at university and fail to understand why their flatmates do not do the washing up or would want to play loud music or go to parties instead of studying! For adults with autism the behaviour of those who do not have autism (neurotypical) can be confusing (Box 9.4).

Thinking and behaviour in autism is often described as inflexible (Box 9.5). Adults with autism prefer rigid routines and dislike change.

The lack of instinctive understanding of others means that the world can seem confusing and unpredictable. Self-imposed predictability adds an element of control and reduces anxiety (Box 9.6).

Change or unpredictable circumstances often unmask difficulties. For some adults with autism not diagnosed in childhood, it is at these points of uncertainty and difficulties in coping that the diagnosis becomes evident. Adults may request assessment for autism after significant and unpredicted events in their lives such as the breakdown of their marriage, loss of job, enforced change to new job in new location or death of a close family member. Although these examples would be difficult for anyone to experience, the impact on someone with autism can be catastrophic.

Even though adults can have good intellectual ability, day-to-day activities such as finding their way to a new appointment or travelling on public transport in rush hour is very daunting.

ABC of Autism, First Edition. Munib Haroon.
© 2019 John Wiley & Sons Ltd. Published 2019 by John Wiley & Sons Ltd.

Box 9.1 **Social interaction can be awkward or unusual – how might an adult with autism present?**

- They may reply to questions but then make no attempt to build on this to keep a to-and-fro conversation going. Alternatively, if the question is of particular interest they may talk at length, be difficult to interrupt and seemingly ignore any non-verbal or verbal cues to end the conversation (as they have not understood the hint)
- The difficulties with social cues means that they may invade personal space or interact in a way that feels over-familiar
- They may not give consistent eye contact – this may be avoidant, fleeting or they may stare intently
- They may have problems with understanding verbal and non-verbal language such that there is/are:
  - incongruent or non-existent facial expressions
  - an unusual tone of voice (monotone or high pitched) or an unexpected accent
  - gestures that seem repetitive and unrelated to the conversation
  - a literal interpretation of what is said and clear difficulty with sarcasm or jokes

Box 9.2 **Features that might prompt a referral for an autism assessment in someone with normal or high intellect**

- Naïve in social situations or inappropriate behaviour or language (over-familiar)
- Pedantic speech and poor non-verbal communication (exaggerated or limited gestures)
- Clumsy, odd posture
- Appears to lack common sense despite intellectual ability
- Apparent lack of empathy and difficulty understanding social cues
- Inflexible routines and thinking
- Eccentricities including all absorbing interests – can be related to work or academic interests
- Strong sense of right and wrong
- Misunderstood, history of bullying – low self-esteem
- Sensitive to criticism

Box 9.3 **Case vignette: Mary**

In the absence of instinctive understanding of how to behave, adults with autism mimic those around them.

Mary was admitted to an elderly psychiatry ward after the sudden death of her parents resulted in challenging behaviours. She immediately began to copy the behaviour of those around her in her new environment which led to an incorrect diagnosis of dementia. She now lives in a home that specialises in caring for adults with autism.

Box 9.4 **Neurotypical world**

The neurotypical world can be confusing and peculiar and autistic adults can perceive that those who do not have autism behave in a way that is difficult to understand
  Neurotypical adults:
- Do not always do what they say they will do
- Can change plans and their minds about things
- Are irrational in their actions, feelings and thoughts
- Make conclusions based on intuition or bits of information, and half-finished sentences
- Use implied vocal and gestural signals
- Prefer to talk about themselves, feelings and relationships rather than factual information
- Use non-verbal and non-literal communication

Box 9.5 **Inflexible thinking and behaviour**

Adults with autism:
- Have difficulty understanding and predicting other people's intentions and behaviour
- Are unable to imagine social situations that are outside their own routine and cannot predict what might happen
- Develop routines and repetitive behaviours to help them cope with the complexity, novelty and messiness of everyday life
- Develop extreme distress (sometimes termed catastrophic rage or meltdowns) if the event is significant and unexpected

Box 9.6 **Examples of self-imposed predictability**

What to look out for in general interview:
- Avoiding crowded places such as large shopping centres
- Narrow deep interests (e.g. may forget to eat when absorbed)
- Preference for repetition and routine – shopping for the same things at the same time in the same place
- Preference for predictability/clarity/order – knowing exactly what is happening, repeatedly asking for confirmation of appointments, wanting very specific information
- Difficulties multitasking – only able to do one thing at a time
- Change causing anxiety
- Attention to detail
- Stereotyped and repetitive behaviours
- Compulsive routines (but no sense that these are inappropriate) and unusual attachments

When considering a diagnosis of autism in adulthood, it is important to collate current clinical evidence of deficits in communication (Boxes 9.7 and 9.8) and social interaction (Box 9.9) across a range of contexts and repetitive and restricted patterns of behaviour, interest or activities (Boxes 9.2, 9.5 and 9.6). Symptoms must have been present from childhood and cause current significant impairment in important areas of their life such as socially or at work.

Some of the language anomalies described in Box 9.8 are important as they can often sound like a thought disorder, and if you add in the use of the third person when some people refer to themselves (this may be mistaken for hallucinatory experiences), a psychotic disorder may be wrongly suspected.

In the most recent update of autism classification (DSM-5), the presence of unusual sensory issues (which has been well known to

Box 9.7 **Difficulty using and understanding verbal and non-verbal language**

- **Gestures** may be over-exaggerated, not in keeping with the content of the conversation or very limited/absent
- **Social gaze** is often unusual. The classic absence of eye contact in childhood is often missing in adulthood, because of the repeated instructions from parents or teachers 'to look at people when talking to them', but the quality of eye contact may be unusual – fleeting or unusually even (because of lack of social instinct some people time or count how long they hold the gaze and then look away as they cannot work this out naturally)
- **Facial expressions** may be incongruous – smiling or laughing when telling a sad story, or a fixed grin or an expression that gives no indication of how they are feeling
- **Tone of voice** may be monotonous, of unusual pitch (high or low) or the person may speak with an American accent (learnt from Disney Films) despite living in the UK
- **Jokes** Difficulty understanding humour unless it is slapstick – may try out jokes in inappropriate settings which can be misconstrued as racist or sexist, etc.
- **Sarcasm and irony** are often difficult to understand and may be taken literally. The literal interpretation of things can also cause problems. An employer suggesting sarcastically that someone might as well go home if that is the type of work they are going to do would not expect them to leave the premises!
- **None or fairly limited speech** Some choose not to communicate using speech or have little usable speech. In these circumstances, never underestimate how much they understand – just because they do not speak does not mean they do not understand exactly what you are saying

Box 9.8 **Some language difficulties that can be seen in an adult with autism**

- **Abnormal prosody** The normal up and down modulation and tone of voice can be much more computer-like and mechanical. In some cases, language and phrases have been learnt from TV and films and therefore the accent can seem incongruent and unexpected given their heritage
- **Language development** The history in the medical notes may suggest deviant or delayed language or conversely unimpaired or even advanced language development. In adulthood, there can be language problems but even where language is not delayed, the use of speech does not seem normal (e.g. using abnormally complex language when the situation does not demand it or making repeated subtle grammatical errors out of keeping with intellectual ability)
- **Echolalia** is the repetition of speech. It may be subtle – the autistic person merely repeating the last couple of words that have been said, as if in acknowledgement. This can be accompanied by **echopraxia** where the adult is copying the gestures or actions of the person interacting with them
- **Pronominal reversal** Autistic adults can have difficulty using pronouns correctly when referring to themselves (e.g. using he or she instead of I)
- **Use of third person** Autistic adults may refer to themselves in the third person, using their own name when talking about themselves. Research suggests this may not just be a language issue, but could be related to the concept of self
- **Other language anomalies** There are many similarities with speech disorder seen in mental health conditions such as schizophrenia which can cause confusion and incorrect diagnosis. Adults with autism may use their own jargon or idiosyncratic and unusual terms (neologisms). The speech may be tangential, verbose and circumstantial (extremely long winded and difficult to follow) and they may verbalise every thought (running commentary)

Box 9.9 **Examples of problems with social interaction**

- Lack of social relationships. It may have been hard to make friends and keep them. In clinic ask about friendships at school and college – have they kept in touch – do they have friends now that they meet (including online friends)?
- Often seems to be a history of bullying at school
- Difficulty with social cues – tendency to stand too close, keep talking when the listener is clearly not interested or trying to leave, preferring to be alone
- Difficulty understanding and predicting other people's intentions and behaviour
- Cannot imagine situations that are outside their own routine – lack social imagination (but female adults especially may be very creative)
- Difficulty recognising and understanding other people's feelings and managing their own feelings
- Cause offence without intention because of a lack of understanding (e.g. if someone asks their opinion on an outfit, they tell the truth). It is important to note that adults, especially women, with autism may have learnt not to give an opinion when asked so no longer make faux pas
- Failure to recognise emotional cues – do not notice when someone is upset and do not provide comfort, not because of a lack of caring, but a lack of awareness of what to do
- Impaired expression or response – laugh at sad news
- Impaired interpretation of a situation
- Problems with personal organisation and time management can also impact on social relationships

Box 9.10 **Sensory issues**

- **Hypo- or hypersensitive hearing** – can hear a conversation in another room. Be careful not to confuse this with auditory hallucinations
- **Hypo- or hypersensitivity to pain** – may not present with significant pathology until very late or, in contrast, may scream in agony if someone brushed past them lightly in a crowd
- **Hypo- or hypersensitivity to light** – may wear dark glasses, or make work colleagues sit in the dark as the fluorescent bulb makes a buzzing noise and flickers
- **Hypo- or hypersensitivity to touch** – at the extreme may not be able to tolerate the sensation of clothing, or may choose the entire wardrobe based on how it feels or cut all the labels from T-shirts or shirts

clinicians for many years) has been acknowledged and added to the diagnostic criteria. Of course, it is possible to have hypo- or hypersensitivity and not be autistic, but it is worth considering sensory issues as they can have a large impact on the presentation (Box 9.10).

Summary

In addition to social interaction, social communication difficulties and restricted, repetitive patterns of behaviour, interests and activities, do not forget that autism is a neurodevelopmental condition whose core features can present in a very variable way and which can also be associated with a number of co-morbid features and associated disorders.

Further reading

National Institute for Health and Clinical Excellence (NICE). Autism spectrum guidance in adults: diagnosis and management. NICE Guideline CG142. London: NICE, 2012 (updated 2016). Available from: https://www.nice.org.uk/guidance/cg142. Accessed: 19 November 2018.

CHAPTER 10

The Assessment and Diagnosis of Autism in Adults

Alison Stansfield

OVERVIEW

- Autism is a developmental condition which may not be diagnosed until adulthood.
- The prevalence in adults in England is over 1%.
- The Autism Act 2009 enshrines in law statutory guidance for health and social care organisations for England and Wales.
- For adults with undetected autism, there are many benefits to acquiring a diagnosis in adulthood.
- Diagnosis in adulthood can prove complicated and requires a comprehensive assessment by a competent, trained, multidisciplinary team.
- Particular tools are used to assist diagnosis but are not in themselves diagnostic.
- This final diagnostic decision is a clinical one and should be based on:
  - a high quality developmental history with collateral information
  - current clinical evidence of deficits in communication and social interaction across a range of settings
  - the presence of restricted, repetitive patterns of behaviour, interests or activities.

Autism is a developmental condition, meaning that it originates in childhood and therefore should be diagnosed in childhood. In reality, this depends on the opportunities for recognition and available resources, and so diagnosis can be missed in childhood for a variety of reasons (Box 10.1).

This delay or lack of diagnosis historically means that accurate information about the prevalence of autism has been difficult to ascertain. Originally, prevalence rates were based on studies in childhood, but a standardised, whole population sample, case-finding study published in December 2016 confirmed the combined prevalence of autism in adults of all ages in England was 11/1000 (i.e. 1.1%).

Autism prevalence rates appear to have increased over time for a number of possible reasons (Box 10.2).

In England and Wales in 2009, it became easier to access diagnostic services in adulthood because of the Autism Act 2009. This stated that the government had to produce a strategy for adults with autism (March 2010) along with statutory guidance for local councils and local health bodies on implementing the strategy (December 2010). Updates have been produced in 2014 and 2015, respectively (Box 10.3). These documents state that adults should be able to access a diagnostic assessment, obtain support if they need it and have services treat them fairly and as individuals (Box 10.4).

Why is it important that adults with autism, not diagnosed in childhood, access autism assessments as adults?

For some adults, autism does not cause them significant problems because of robust protective factors such as a secure and protected working environment (e.g. academic institution), an understanding and supportive social/family network and/or learnt social adaptations. However, for others, autism can contribute to significant ongoing difficulties in both health and social (including occupational, educational and accommodation) arenas.

Although recognition of autism in childhood to address needs earlier in life is preferable, diagnosis in adulthood can be extremely beneficial. This is evidenced by feedback from autistic people who have received a diagnosis in adulthood in Leeds (Leeds Autism Diagnostic Service, LADS; Box 10.5).

The Autism Act 2009 states that the NHS has a duty to provide diagnostic assessments for autism in adulthood but is less prescriptive about post-diagnostic support. There is a huge disparity in the support available for adults diagnosed with autism compared to those who were diagnosed in childhood, although this is improving.

In August 2017, NICE recommended that GPs record when someone has received a diagnosis of autism.

ABC of Autism, First Edition. Munib Haroon.
© 2019 John Wiley & Sons Ltd. Published 2019 by John Wiley & Sons Ltd.

Box 10.1 Possible reasons for failure to diagnose autism in childhood

- Inadequate resources (child psychiatry/paediatric expertise)
- Other difficulties within the family/child which override concerns about autism (e.g. extremely difficult behaviour or childhood abuse)
- Co-morbidities (e.g. learning disabilities, anxiety, OCD, genetic conditions)
- Symptoms do not cause a problem in childhood (e.g. 'easy baby'; impeccably behaved, high achieving student)
- Child shares similar characteristics with their family
- Child develops coping strategies that hide their social difficulties

Box 10.2 Reasons for changes in prevalence

- Change in diagnostic understanding of autism as a spectrum
- Greater awareness
- Improved recognition
- Improved training
- Autism specific diagnostic services for children *and* adults

Box 10.3 The Autism Act 2009

First ever disability-specific legislation to be passed in the UK
Led to the publication of:
- 'Fulfilling and rewarding lives' – the strategy for adults with autism in England March 2010
- Statutory Guidance – Implementing 'Fulfilling and rewarding lives' December 2010
- 'Fulfilling and rewarding lives' – the strategy for adults with autism in England, an update 2014 (Think Autism)
- Statutory guidance for local authorities and NHS organisations to support implementation of the Adult Autism Strategy 2015
- Think Autism strategy: governance refresh 2018

Box 10.4 What does The Autism Act say?

'All adults with autism are able to live fulfilling and rewarding lives within a society that accepts and understands them, they can get a diagnosis and access support if they need it, and they can depend on mainstream public services to treat them fairly as individuals, helping them make the most of their talents'

Diagnosis in adulthood

Following the Autism Act, autism diagnostic services were set up across England and Wales. Services vary according to the expertise and background of local clinicians, variations in funding, resources and commissioning arrangements. There is ongoing work to capture the differences in adult autism diagnostic provision in England and Wales.

Box 10.5 Why is it important that adults with autism, not diagnosed in childhood, access autism assessments as adults?

- Validates long-standing feelings of being different and not fitting in
- Helps work colleagues/employees and academic institutions to tolerate and make reasonable adjustments to their idiosyncrasies
- Enables the person to be appointed because of their personal understanding of autism for employment as an advisor to health and social care
- Facilitates access to an autism alert card for use in times of crisis when communication and expression of need is most difficult. (An alert card is credit card sized and states that the person carrying it has autism and usually includes an explanatory leaflet about autism)
- Enables a social care assessment which highlights unmet needs and access to benefits and resources including accommodation, education and occupation and ultimately better integration into the community
- For many, a missed autism diagnosis leads to a series of inaccurate and unnecessary mental health labels or, conversely, the development of mental health co-morbidities (see Chapter 11)
- May allow diversion from hospital, the court or prison

Diagnostic classification systems and guides for autism

As in childhood, there are two international classification systems used for diagnosing autism in adults: DSM-5 and ICD-10 (see Chapter 2), and two UK specific current guidelines for diagnosing autism in adulthood (Box 10.6).

How to diagnose autism in adulthood

Even when the person being assessed is an adult, diagnosis is still based on the establishment of a good developmental history relating to childhood as well as **current** clinical evidence. The exact diagnostic assessment process for different services will vary but there are likely to be many similarities.

A comprehensive diagnostic assessment should be undertaken by competent trained staff as part of a multidisciplinary team. A series of tools can be used to aid the process (Box 10.7). However,

Box 10.6 Current guidelines for diagnosing autism in adulthood

England

National Institute for Health and Care Excellence (NICE)
NICE Autism spectrum disorder in adults: diagnosis and management. Clinical guideline CG142. Published date: June 2012. Last updated: August 2016

Scotland

Scottish Intercollegiate Guidelines Network (SIGN)
SIGN 145 Assessment, diagnosis and interventions for autism spectrum disorders: a national clinical guideline. June 2016

Box 10.7 **Examples of assessment tools used in an adult autism assessment**

- Autism Diagnostic Interview – Revised (ADI-R)
- Diagnostic Interview for Social and Communication Disorders (DISCO)
- Autism Diagnostic Observation Schedule – Generic (ADOS-G)
- Developmental, Dimensional and Diagnostic Interview (3Di)
- Asperger Syndrome (and high-functioning autism) Diagnostic Interview (ASDI)
- Ritvo Autism Asperger Diagnostic Scale – Revised (RAADS-R)

ultimately the final decision about diagnosis is a clinical one based on a high quality developmental history with, where possible, supporting collateral information from medical, social and school reports and current clinical evidence.

The aim of the diagnostic process is for the multidisciplinary clinicians to collate:

- **Current** clinical evidence of deficits in social communication and social interaction across a range of contexts and restricted, repetitive patterns of behaviour, interest or activities;
- Evidence that symptoms are **developmental** (i.e. present from childhood although may present differently at different stage of life);
- Evidence that symptoms cause **current significant impairment** in important areas of their life (i.e. social or work settings).

As part of the diagnostic process, it is also important that there is an assessment of risks such as: self harm or to others, the risk of exploitation/abuse and disintegration of support. Concerns should be expeditiously escalated when necessary.

It may be helpful to develop a safety plan and consider additional investigations including for the exclusion of other diagnoses.

Service Example: Leeds Autism Diagnostic Service (LADS)

The following is an example of an adult diagnostic service based in Leeds to illustrate the potential journey of an adult being assessed for autism via a recognised integrated pathway.

In Leeds, the diagnostic service is an all IQ service which means that it accepts referrals irrespective of intellectual ability. The team consists of clinicians with expertise in intellectual disability as well as from general adult mental health services. The diagnostic pathway is illustrated in Figure 10.1.

The pathway is an open referral pathway (meaning that anyone can refer, including self-refer). As an initial step, a pack including questionnaires is sent to the person's home. This is returned prior to the first appointment being sent out. The screening assessment is carried out to exclude co-morbidities and risks that need attention, identify an appropriate informant for the developmental interview and request reports/DVDs/photos. The subsequent assessment, which includes a developmental interview, is carried out with the use of standardised tools (e.g. ADI-R or DISCO). The subsequent clinical decisions meeting allows the opportunity for a further interview and for observational assessments (based on ADOS) to be carried out. The final diagnostic decision, which is given at a follow-up appointment, is based on a multidisciplinary clinical consensus incorporating all the developmental and collateral history and clinical observations.

Hurdles during assessment

The available standardised tools to collect developmental information, which are used in adult assessments, were developed for research and specifically for use with children. They can take a significant amount of time to administer (2–7 hours). It is generally accepted by expert clinicians that these tools can provide false positives and negatives, for example in adults with learning disabilities, speech and language disorders and women.

The autism observational assessment (based on the ADOS, which was also developed for use with children) allows the clinicians to observe adults in a less formalised clinical setting but some adults object to being assessed using such childish tools; however, there is currently no recommended adult alternative.

It is important to note that while a developmental history is a crucial part of the assessment, there may be many hurdles to overcome in obtaining it (Box 10.8).

If it is not possible to access a detailed developmental history and the collateral information is limited, the person being referred is told at an early stage that it may not be possible to reach a diagnostic conclusion. Sometimes, people who previously did not want the assessors to talk to their family will agree to allow this as long as the appointments are separated, so they do not have to meet. If the relatives live in a different country they may agree to an interview being sent by email, or undertaken on the telephone.

In cases where parents or close family have died or have no contact and school reports have been destroyed, then a degree of 'thinking outside the box' to obtain a broader perspective on the person's presentation is required (Box 10.9).

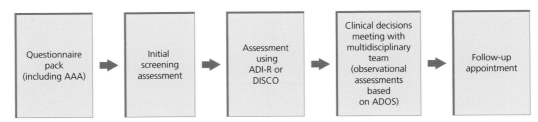

Figure 10.1 Example of diagnostic pathway in Leeds: Leeds Autism Diagnostic Pathway (LADS).

Box 10.8 **Hurdles to accessing a detailed developmental history in adulthood**

- Lack of informants, for example if the person being referred has no living relatives, or has relatives who live in another country
- The person does not want their relatives to know about the assessment, usually because family members have been negative about such an assessment
- The person does not want their relatives to be contacted because of a family history of sexual or other types of abuse
- There has been a family dispute and they are no longer in contact with family members
- School reports have been lost or destroyed

Box 10.9 **Thinking outside the box to get collateral and current observational information**

- Meeting for a coffee in a coffee shop enables observation of social interaction in a less clinical setting
- Talking to current employers, colleagues or academic tutors can provide a very different perspective
- Talking to friends and associates of current special interest groups (e.g. amateur dramatics) who meet the person on a regular basis due to the shared interest

Autism assessment in adults may need to involve a degree of innovative thinking to give the adult the best chance of receiving a valid and relevant diagnosis that at the very least enables them to understand themselves better and at best facilitates access to supports that enable a fulfilling and rewarding life.

Further reading

Autism Act 2009. Available from: http://www.legislation.gov.uk/ukpga/2009/15/contents. Accessed: 20 November 2018.

Brugha T, Spiers N, Bankart J, Cooper S. Epidemiology of autism in adults across age groups and ability levels. British Journal of Psychiatry 2016; 209: 498–503.

National Institute for Health and Clinical Excellence (NICE). Autism spectrum guidance in adults: diagnosis and management. NICE guideline CG142. London: NICE, 2012 (updated 2016). Available from: https://www.nice.org.uk/guidance/cg142. Accessed: 20 November 2018.

Scottish Intercollegiate Guidelines Network (SIGN). Assessment, diagnosis and interventions for autism spectrum disorders. SIGN publication no. 145. Edinburgh: SIGN, 2016. Available from: http://sign.ac.uk. Accessed: 20 November 2018.

CHAPTER 11

Autism and Mental Health in Adult Patients

Conor Davidson

OVERVIEW

- Mental health problems are very often seen in adults with autism.
- The most common co-morbidities are anxiety disorders, depression and ADHD.
- Assessment of mental state can be more challenging in patients with autism. Consider the timescale of the symptoms and carefully examine non-verbal communication.
- Psychiatric treatment is generally effective for co-morbid mental health problems in autism, but sometimes adaptations are required.

People with autism are more susceptible to mental health problems than neurotypicals. This is for a variety of reasons: genetic vulnerability, communication difficulties, problems with jobs or relationships, and so on. (Box 11.1). It is estimated that over half of all adults with autism will also have at least one other diagnosable mental health condition. Even for those autistic people who do not meet the clinical threshold for a co-morbid mental health disorder, it is very common to feel demoralised and exhausted by the daily struggle to cope with and understand the neurotypical world.

Clinicians working in all settings will come across autistic patients. Given the high rates of mental health problems in this group, it is important to be able to recognise and if necessary treat co-morbid psychiatric symptoms. A common misconception in the past was that conventional psychiatric treatments do not work for people with autism. By and large this is not the case, although some treatments (particularly psychotherapies) can require some modification. Unfortunately, awareness and understanding of autism is still not always as good as it could be amongst mental health professionals – particularly in working age adult services who historically have viewed autism as 'not core business' – but thankfully this attitude is gradually changing. The presence of autism should never be used as a justification for denying access to a service or treatment. All health services should be prepared to make reasonable adjustments to optimise care to autistic people, and these kinds of adjustments will benefit all their patients.

Assessment of mental state

The elements of a standard mental state examination are shown in Box 11.2.

Autism can cause abnormalities in many of these domains and mimic other psychiatric conditions, potentially causing confusion to the uninitiated examiner. Common findings are as follows.

- **Appearance and behaviour** People with autism are often less concerned about conforming to social norms; therefore their dress, appearance and behaviour can appear odd or unusual. Examples we have seen in clinic include: always wearing the same outfit every day, wearing clothes inappropriate to the season (e.g. sandals in winter) and only wearing clothes of a certain colour or fabric (often related to sensory sensitivity). Gender fluidity is more common. Behaviour can appear socially disinhibited or even bizarre (e.g. sitting facing away from the examiner). There may be repetitive movements (e.g. hand wringing, rocking) or tics.
- **Speech** Often odd or unusual in autism. It can be abnormal in volume, tone or rate. The accent may be strange. We have seen a number of patients with American accents despite never having set foot in the USA, presumably because of the influence of movies and TV. Poverty of speech (i.e. not talking much) can be seen, as can pressured speech (talking too much). There is less reciprocity to the conversation – it can feel like the patient is talking 'at' you rather than 'with' you.
- **Mood** Affect can be restricted (i.e. less range of facial expression) or incongruous (e.g. smiling at a sad story). Anxiety and nervousness is common, particularly in the clinic setting. People with autism can struggle to access or describe their inner emotional states (more so if they also have learning disability), so may not be able to self-report low or elevated mood.
- **Thought form** Sometimes this is repetitive and hard to follow: 'on a different wavelength' to the interviewer.
- **Thought content** People with autism can be fixed on one theme (special interest).
- **Perception** The person with autism may take questions literally. For example, when asked 'do you hear voices', they reply 'yes',

when in fact they can hear the interviewer's voice. Autistic people often have sensory differences, which can manifest as either hyper- or hyposensitivity in any sensory domain.

- **Insight** Some patients lack insight about having autism. They can also be more prone to lacking insight into other psychiatric conditions.
- **Cognition** Learning disability, attention deficit and impaired (social) judgement are all more common.

So how to cut through the confusion? When taking a psychiatric history from a patient with autism (or suspected autism), take care to use clear, unambiguous language. Check for understanding and clarify your meaning if necessary. Observe the timescales carefully – by definition, features of autism will be present in childhood, whereas most mental illnesses first present in adolescence or adulthood. A collateral history from an informant who knew the patient as a child is invaluable. When conducting a mental state examination, pay close attention to non-verbal communication.

Because patients with autism can have an odd communication style, and repetitive or unusual behaviours, it is very helpful if the assessing clinician has some prior knowledge of the patient. If there is a change from the normal pattern of behaviour, it may be indicative of a mental disorder.

Transitions

Certain times of a person's life can be particularly difficult, and this is especially the case for people with autism; this includes leaving school and going to college. These types of major life changes can increase the risk of mental health problems developing.

The next section looks at individual mental disorders and their relation to autism.

Other developmental disorders

Developmental disorders tend to cluster together and overlap. It is estimated that 25% of people with autism also have ADHD. Consider the possibility of co-morbid ADHD whenever there are prominent symptoms of inattention, hyperactivity and impulsivity. Bear in mind that mood instability is very commonly seen in ADHD, which can be mistaken for bipolar disorder or emotionally unstable personality disorder.

Tics are present in 10% of autistic patients, Tourette's syndrome in 5%. Dyspraxia (developmental coordination disorder) is also common. Patients with autism will often report a long history of physical clumsiness. They may also walk with a stiff or unusual gait.

Anxiety disorders

Any clinician working with autistic adults will observe high rates of anxiety. About 40% of adults with autism, according to some data, will have a clinically diagnosable anxiety disorder. Some patients first present with an anxiety problem, which later leads to a diagnosis of autism. The two most common anxiety disorders seen in autism are social phobia and generalised anxiety disorder. The pattern of anxiety and triggering factors will differ from person to person, but some commonly seen triggers are listed in Box 11.3. Increased levels of anxiety typically result in increased levels of repetitive behaviour, or increased preoccupation with special interests. Anxiety can present dramatically with 'meltdowns' involving shouting, swearing, damage to property or aggression.

Obsessive compulsive disorder

Repetitive behaviours are often seen in autism, but it is important to distinguish these from clinical obsessive compulsive disorder (OCD) (Table 11.1). Probably the most crucial difference is that in

Table 11.1 Key differences between repetitive behaviours in autism and OCD.

Autism	OCD
Compulsions (restricted and repetitive behaviours)	Obsessions + compulsions
Egosyntonic	Egodystonic
Hoarding, repeating, reordering	Contamination, aggressive/sexual thoughts, checking
Rarely seek treatment	Often seek treatment
Less likely to respond to SSRI antidepressants	More likely to respond to SSRIs

OCD the obsessions and compulsions are experienced by the patient as unpleasant, intrusive and irrational (egodystonic), whereas repetitive behaviours in autism are generally soothing and pleasant (egosyntonic).

True OCD can occur in autism, indeed it is at least twice as common as in the general population. It is still important to distinguish carefully between wanted and unwanted thoughts and behaviours. It is pointless to attempt to 'treat' a repetitive behaviour that the patient in fact finds soothing.

Depression

A degree of low mood is very common in adult patients seen in clinic. Patients complain of 'not fitting in', a sense that 'something isn't quite right' or feeling exhausted and overwhelmed by the demands of life. The prevalence of clinical depression (major depressive disorder) is in the order of 30%. Some patients with autism will have difficulty accessing or describing their internal mood state, so depression may be most evident through change in behaviour –more social withdrawal, increase (or decrease) in repetitive behaviour, irritability, change in sleep or eating pattern. Psychotic depression can occur. Catatonia appears to be more common.

Risk of suicide is important. A recent study found that 66% of adults with Asperger's syndrome had suicidal thoughts, compared with 17% of the general population. Elevated rates of death by suicide contribute to the excess mortality in people with autism, who on average die 16 years younger than the general population.

Bipolar affective disorder

Bipolar disorder appears to be more common in adults with autism. Care must be taken over diagnosis. Some autistic people habitually talk rapidly without pause, with little regard to social niceties and this can be mistaken for the pressure of speech and social disinhibition of mania. Sleep disturbance and mood changes are also frequently seen in autism but are not necessarily indicative of bipolar disorder. The key thing to establish is 'what is this patient's normal presentation?'

When manic states occur in people with autism, they can be characterised by social withdrawal and self-neglect. The patient will have decreased need for sleep and increased motor activation, but overactivity can be directed at repetitive behaviours, special interests or other relatively narrow pursuits.

Psychotic disorders

Psychosis is a state of disconnection from reality characterised by delusions and hallucinations. Psychotic states can occur in the context of almost any psychiatric disorder. Schizophrenia is the paradigmatic psychotic disorder, in which recurrent episodes of psychosis are accompanied by disorganised thoughts and behaviours, and where 'negative symptoms' accumulate over time. Negative symptoms include blunted affect, lack of energy/motivation, and poverty of speech. Clinically, it is often difficult to distinguish chronic schizophrenia from autism in older adults (Box 11.4) – careful

---

Box 11.4 A case example illustrating the diagnostic challenges in older adults

Case example: schizophrenia or autism?

This 54-year-old man had lived with his mother all his life and was heavily dependent on her for nearly all day-to-day tasks. He had been shy throughout childhood and was bullied at school. He found it difficult to make friends, and had never had a sexual partner.

He had an intense interest in trains and spent all his spare cash on model trains and tracks. He photographed trains and had numerous books and magazines about them.

As a young man he had worked in semi-skilled mechanical jobs on trains and cars. At the age of 25 he lost his job and became even more reliant on his parents. He began suffering from low mood, 'bizarre behaviour' (buying random objects on impulse, running away from home, ducking down in shops) and became paranoid about going outside.

He was admitted to a psychiatric inpatient ward and subsequently a day hospital. On assessment he was judged to be suffering from thought disorder and paranoid thinking. Later on (presumably after being asked about auditory hallucinations multiple times) he said he was hearing 'muffled voices' talking to him, and was diagnosed with schizophrenia.

For nearly 20 years he was treated with a variety of antipsychotics until 10 years ago he decided to stop taking them. This made no appreciable difference to his presentation.

Table 11.2 Key clinical differences between autism and schizophrenia.

Autism	Schizophrenia
Features apparent from early childhood	Onset not until adolescence or later
No hallucinations or delusions	Hallucinations and delusions prominent
Features of autism tend to be fixed over time	Often a relapsing and remitting course
Little response to antipsychotic medication beyond a non-specific calming effect	Specific response to antipsychotic medication in most cases

examination of the course and onset of illness is crucial in these cases. The key differences are shown in Table 11.2.

There is little agreement in the literature about the true rate of co-morbidity of autism and schizophrenia. Certainly, autism is not protective from schizophrenia, and it may even predispose. Individuals with autism and learning disability are less likely to be diagnosed with schizophrenia than higher functioning autistic people, perhaps because poor verbal ability makes diagnosis more difficult. There is a recognised association between Asperger's syndrome and brief and transient (cycloid) psychosis.

Personality disorders

The concept of personality disorder is arguably the least reliable and least valid in all of psychiatry. The diagnostic rubric for personality disorders is likely to be significantly revised in ICD-11. Currently, they are broadly divided into cluster A (odd, eccentric), cluster B (dramatic, erratic) and cluster C (anxious, fearful). The defining feature of all personality disorders is difficulty relating to other people. Some experts in the field argue that schizoid personality disorder (solitary, detached, anhedonic) is in fact a variant of autism. Patients with personality disorder often score highly on questionnaires of autistic traits, and often exhibit abnormal responses in the ADOS.

These caveats notwithstanding, in our clinical experience it is generally possible to distinguish between personality disorder and autism. The age of onset of personality disorder is generally in adolescence or early adulthood, as opposed to the childhood onset of autism. Although personality disorder is characterised by difficulties in relationships with others, social instinct tends to be preserved (the patient knows how they *should* behave, but is unable or unwilling to do so). Patients with personality disorder usually – but not always – report a history of childhood abuse or neglect. Repeated self-harm is more commonly seen in personality disorder than autism.

The question arises, what does co-morbid autism and personality disorder look like? There is little consensus on this. It should be considered whenever a patient presents with clear childhood onset of autistic features, but also with significant problems regulating emotions and behaviour from adolescence onwards. In these cases the presence of childhood trauma can be a major confounding factor and can make drawing firm conclusions regarding diagnosis very difficult.

Substance misuse

Several studies have reported that drug and alcohol use is lower amongst autistic adolescents than in age-matched neurotypical peers. This is thought to be because of the reduced effect of peer influence (put bluntly, teenagers with autism may not get invited to the sorts of parties where drinking and drug-taking goes on). Perhaps there is also an element of rigid adherence to rules – 'underage drinking is illegal therefore I can't do it' – or non-conformity. It has also been suggested that people with autism have reduced pleasurable effects from alcohol. As they enter adulthood, the differences in substance use between autistic people and neurotypicals become less pronounced. Adults with autism may drink or take drugs in order to reduce anxiety, to boost mood or to try and 'fit in' with others.

Treatment considerations

There are currently no proven effective treatments for the core symptoms of autism. However, mental health co-morbidities can be effectively treated in most cases. There are certain considerations and adjustments that should be taken into account.

Antidepressants
Selective serotonin reuptake inhibitors (SSRIs) are regarded as the first line treatment for anxiety and depression in autism. They can also be of benefit for troublesome repetitive behaviours and obsessional symptoms. Some studies suggest that people with autism are more sensitive to side effects, in particular behavioural overactivation, from SSRIs. It is prudent to start on the lowest possible dose and allow at least 4 weeks before cautiously increasing dosage.

Antipsychotics
The most widely studied antipsychotic in autism is risperidone. Risperidone is commonly used to treat challenging behaviour in autism, but it is also an effective antipsychotic. Alternatives include olanzapine or aripiprazole. Aripiprazole is particularly useful when weight gain or sedation is a problem. People with autism appear to be sensitive to antipsychotic side effects, including motor side effects like stiffness, tremor and – in extremis – catatonia. Again, only the lowest effective dosage should be used. Response should be carefully monitored; as brief and transient psychosis is more common in autism, duration of antipsychotic treatment may need to be shorter than normal.

Psychological therapy
Cognitive behavioural therapy (CBT) is a safe and effective treatment for a wide range of anxiety and depressive disorders. People with autism tend to do well with CBT, but certain adaptations may need to be made: for instance: shorter sessions, highly structured, clear goals and more emphasis on behavioural strategies rather than cognitive analysis. More highly analytical forms of psychological therapy, such as psychodynamic therapy or cognitive analytical therapy, may not be as effective. People with autism usually have a concrete thinking style and can have difficulty grasping the more abstract concepts involved in these types of therapies.

Social interventions
Many people with autism feel like strangers in a strange world. They feel like they do not fit in. Finding a role and purpose in life can be key to improving mental well-being. For instance, getting a job where the person's autistic traits are celebrated and valued (e.g. work requiring a great deal of focus and attention to detail). Health professionals can help by guiding the patient to appropriate autism support services in the local community. The National Autistic Society is a good source of information.

Reasonable adjustments
Going to see a health professional for the first time can be daunting and anxiety-provoking for someone with autism. It involves a deviation from normal routine, meeting a new person in an unfamiliar place, and a high degree of social interaction. The Equality Act 2010 requires services to make 'reasonable adjustments' for people with a disability, including autism. There are reasonable adjustments that can be considered in the primary care setting (Box 11.5).

Interface between primary and secondary care

There is a well-recognised problem with adults with autism 'falling through the gaps' in services, particularly higher functioning individuals who are not eligible for learning disability services. Autism has traditionally not been regarded as part of the 'core business' of secondary mental health services, and it is not unheard of for community mental health teams to resist seeing patients with autism. The UK government Adult Autism Strategy 2010 is very clear that people with autism should not be discriminated against in terms of fair and equitable access to health services.

Box 11.5 **Reasonable adjustments for patients with autism**

Appointments	Offer the first appointment of the day (so the patient is not sitting in a busy waiting room)
	Start and finish the appointment at the expected time
Communication	Use clear, straightforward language
	Write the key points down for the patient to take away
Environment	Walls and other surfaces painted in neutral colours
	Reduce ambient noise and bright lighting as much as possible

---

Box 11.6 **Circumstances that might warrant referral to secondary care mental health services**

- Major mental disorder (e.g. psychotic episode)
- Common mental disorder that is unresponsive to primary care-level treatment (e.g. depression uncontrolled by antidepressant, anxiety disorder not helped by a course of CBT)
- Significant behaviour that challenges (e.g. aggression toward caregivers)
- Significant risk (e.g. suicide attempts)
- Issues requiring expertise in mental health legislation (e.g. Mental Health Act, Mental Capacity Act)

In general, primary care practitioners should follow the same 'stepped care' approach to patients with autism as they do with other patients, but have a lower threshold for each step (as the presence of autism increases complexity). Examples of circumstances in which a referral to secondary mental health services should be considered are shown in Box 11.6.

Use of the Mental Health Act

Autism is considered a 'mental disorder' for the purposes of the Mental Health Act. However, in practice it is unusual to detain an autistic person under the Mental Health Act in the absence of significant co-morbid mental illness. The exception is when the patient is engaging in very challenging or risky behaviour involving aggression or self-harm. Detention in hospital for long periods is generally not helpful for patients with autism, as it is an unfamiliar and high-stimulus environment. Any admission should be kept as short as possible, and alternative community arrangements actively sought.

Further reading

Berney, T. Asperger syndrome from childhood into adulthood. Advances in Psychiatric Treatment 2004; 10: 341–351.

Cassidy S, Bradley P, Robinson J, et al. Suicidal ideation and suicide plans or attempts in adults with Asperger's syndrome attending a specialist diagnostic clinic: a clinical cohort study. Lancet Psychiatry 2014; 1: 142–147.

Equality Act 2010. London: The Stationery Office.

Ghaziuddin, M. Mental Health Aspects of Autism and Asperger Syndrome. London and Philadelphia: Jessica Kingsley, 2005.

Howlin, P. Outcome in adult life for more able individuals with autism or Asperger syndrome. Autism 2000; 4; 63–83.

McDougle C, Kresch L, Goodman WK. Naylor ST. A case–control study of repetitive thoughts and behaviour in adults with autistic disorder and obsessive-compulsive disorder. American Journal of Psychiatry 1995; 152: 772–777.

Royal College of Psychiatrists. Good practice in the management of autism (including Asperger syndrome) in adults. College Report CR191. London: RCPsych, 2014.

Skokauskasa N, Gallagher L. Psychosis, affective disorders and anxiety in autistic spectrum disorder: prevalence and nosological considerations. Psychopathology 2010; 43: 8–16.

Tantam, D. Asperger's syndrome. Journal of Child Psychology and Psychiatry 1988; 29: 245–253.

CHAPTER 12

Learning Disabilities and Autism

Keri-Michele Lodge, Alwyn Kam, and Alison Stansfield

OVERVIEW

- Half of people with autism have a co-morbid learning disability.
- People with autism and a learning disability have complex health needs with implications for morbidity and mortality.
- Health problems present atypically in this population because of communication difficulties and differing perceptions of pain.
- Awareness of common co-morbidities aids clinical detection.
- Health care services must make reasonable adjustments to facilitate access to diagnosis, investigations, treatment and care.
- Reducing the use of inappropriate psychotropic medication is a key priority for this population.

As described in Chapter 10, autism affects people of all intellectual abilities. Although many people with autism are of normal or higher than average intelligence, approximately 50% also have a learning disability (LD). Among people with LD, 30–40% have co-morbid autism (Figure 12.1).

What is a learning disability?

The term 'learning disability', used in the UK, has been superseded by 'intellectual disability' in many countries, replacing more demeaning descriptors used in the past such as 'mental subnormality', 'mental handicap' and 'mental retardation'. A learning disability is not the same as a learning difficulty although the terms are frequently used interchangeable on a day-to-day basis (Box 12.1).

LD is characterised by three core features:

1 Reduced ability to understand new or complex information, or to learn new skills (impaired intelligence with an intelligence quotient (IQ) under 70);
2 Reduced ability to cope with everyday tasks independently (impaired adaptive functioning);
3 Onset before the age of 18, with a lasting effect on development.

A person's intelligence can be assessed using IQ tests, giving an indication of the severity of their learning disability and an estimate of their likely level of functioning (Table 12.1).

Aetiology of learning disability and autism

Although the aetiology of co-morbid autism spectrum disorder (ASD) and LD is incompletely understood, particular factors may be more strongly associated with developing ASD alone, LD alone, or both (Table 12.2).

ASD and LD can occur in a number of genetic syndromes as part of a behavioural phenotype – distinct patterns of behavioural, psychological, emotional, psychiatric and cognitive functioning. Notable examples of such syndromes include Angelman's, Cornelia de Lange, Down's, fragile X, Prader–Willi and Rett's syndromes. Recognising the presence of such syndrome facilitates monitoring for associated co-morbidities, for example, hypothyroidism in people with Down's syndrome. Identifying such syndromes can also benefit families (Box 12.2).

Autism in people with a learning disability

Although ASD is common in people with LD, it should not be assumed that it is always present. Someone with even profound or severe LD can show developmentally appropriate social interaction, for example, sharing laughter at blowing bubbles and indicating that they want the activity to be repeated. When someone with a severe or profound LD has co-morbid ASD, they show little interest in interacting with others unless it meets their needs, for example, when they want a drink or the TV channel changing. Diagnosing ASD in people with LD is a specialist task; referral for a specialist autism diagnostic assessment should be prompted by particular features (Box 12.3).

Autism, learning disability and health

People with ASD and/or LD have significant health care needs, with a different pattern of morbidity and mortality from the general population (Boxes 12.4 and 12.5)

Around one-third of early deaths among people with LD could be avoided with the provision of good quality health care. Premature

---

ABC of Autism, First Edition. Munib Haroon.
© 2019 John Wiley & Sons Ltd. Published 2019 by John Wiley & Sons Ltd.

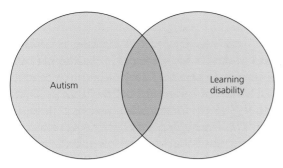

Figure 12.1 Overlap between autism and learning disability.

Box 12.1 What is a learning difficulty?

'Learning difficulty' denotes difficulties with specific abilities used for learning, for example, someone with dyslexia may have difficulties with reading and writing, but, unlike in someone with a learning disability, their overall intelligence and social functioning is not impaired.

Table 12.1 Severity of learning disability.

IQ range	Severity	Level of functioning
50–69	Mild (85% of those with a disability are in the 'mild' range)	Fair language abilities Reasonable level of independence, often able to work Fewer sensory/motor deficits
35–49	Moderate (10% of those with a disability are in the 'moderate' range)	Receptive (understanding others) language often better than expressive (making themselves understood) abilities often require some help with activities of daily living, may be able to work in sheltered employment
20–34	Severe (4% of those with a disability are in the 'severe' range)	Limited communication and limited independence Often live in residential care/nursing care settings Around 50% have epilepsy More severe sensory/motor deficits
<20	Profound (1–2% of those with a disability are in the 'profound' range)	Significant needs. Usually live in residential care/nursing settings with constant supervision Very limited communication, mobility and self-care skills Often have co-morbid hearing and/or visual impairment

Table 12.2 Aetiological factors in autism and learning disability.

	Associated aetiological factors
Autism with learning disability	Poor fetal growth Underlying genetic syndromes
Autism without learning disability	Maternal infection Placental infection
Learning disability without autism	Maternal diabetes Placental abruption

Box 12.2 Benefits to an individual's family of identifying genetic syndromes

- Allows provision of information on the person's likely strengths, needs and prognosis
- Helps families and carers access other sources of support, such as Contact a Family
- Gives families the opportunity to consider genetic counselling

Box 12.3 Learning disability and autism

Consider referral for an autism diagnostic assessment in people with a learning disability with:
- Very limited non-verbal communication (e.g. eye contact, gestures)
- Disinterest in interacting with others except for the purposes of getting needs met
- Clumsy, odd posture
- Extreme anxiety around changes to the environment or their routine (e.g. if their bus is late, or when Christmas decorations are put up)
- Great attention to detail (e.g. picking up tiny pieces of fluff from the carpet)
- Excellent memory
- All-absorbing interests (e.g. flicking or spinning an object for hours)

Box 12.4 Case vignette: Gordon – autism, learning disability and health

Gordon is a 28-year-old man with ASD and LD who cannot speak and lives in a residential care home. His carers take Gordon to see the GP because he has been repeatedly hitting himself on the side of his face. Gordon has not been eating well for a couple of weeks. Gordon is very anxious about going to see the doctor, and becomes distressed in the waiting area, screaming and biting his hand. What would you do?

Box 12.5 Learning disability, autism and mortality

- People with LD in the UK die on average 16 years earlier than those in the general population
- People with ASD and LD may die more than 30 years earlier than the general population

deaths among people with ASD and LD reflect the challenges such individuals encounter when accessing health care (Box 12.6).

Recognising health problems in people with ASD and LD is challenging because of the atypical way these present. People with ASD and LD with limited verbal communication may express symptoms such as pain via their behaviour. There is a risk that such behavioural changes are attributed to the individual's ASD and/or LD, rather than considering the possibility of an underlying physical or mental health cause (diagnostic overshadowing).

With any concerns about behaviour, a broad differential diagnosis should be considered (Box 12.7).

Clinicians should consider the possibility of co-morbidities common in people with ASD and/or LD (Table 12.3).

In the UK, annual health checks are used to identify health care needs in this population (Box 12.8). When investigations and/or treatment are necessary, in England and Wales, the Mental Capacity Act (2005) requires clinicians to assess whether the individual has the mental capacity to make a decision to consent to these. When an individual lacks capacity, decisions about these matters should be made in the person's best interests with the involvement of family and carers.

In Great Britain, the Equality Act (2010) places a duty on public services, including health care services, to make reasonable adjustments to ensure they meet the needs of people with ASD and/or LD. Community LD teams and LD liaison nurses within general hospitals support health care services to make reasonable adjustments (Box 12.9).

Autism, learning disability and behaviour which challenges

Some individuals with ASD and LD are described as having behaviour which challenges (Box 12.10), also referred to as 'challenging behaviour'. This is not a medical or psychiatric diagnosis, and describes the behavioural effects of a problem rather than the cause.

Box 12.6 Factors contributing to health inequalities among people with ASD and LD

- Atypical presentation, particularly in those with limited communication or hypo- or hypersensitivity to pain
- Health care services failing to make adjustments to meet the individual's needs
- Families/carers not being listened to
- Problems with coordination of care and information sharing
- Institutional discrimination

Box 12.7 Underlying causes to consider in individuals with autism and/or learning disability presenting with a change in behaviour

- Pain, including dental
- Gastrointestinal problems, particularly constipation, gastro-oesophageal reflux
- Infection – ears, urinary tract, respiratory tract, skin
- Sensory impairments – visual loss (e.g. cataracts), hearing loss (e.g. wax occlusion)
- Mental health problems (e.g. depression)
- Medication side effects
- Social or environmental stressors (e.g. loss of carer/relative/peer, abuse, neglect, boredom)

Box 12.8 Annual health checks

- People aged 14 and over who have moderate, severe or profound LD, or people with a mild LD and other complex health needs, such as ASD, are entitled to an annual health check in primary care
- There are a number of annual health check templates for primary care practitioners to use
- Annual health checks:
  - identify undetected health conditions early
  - ensure the appropriateness of ongoing treatments
  - promote health (e.g. screening and immunisation)

Table 12.3 Common co-morbidities in people with ASD and/or LD.

Co-morbidity	Clinical implications
Dental: predisposal to dental caries because of difficulties maintaining good oral hygiene, increased prevalence of bruxism and difficulties tolerating regular dental check-ups	Refer to a specialist dental service for a programme of gradual desensitisation, or for examination under sedation Refer to community learning disability team for desensitisation around brushing teeth
Gastrointestinal: increased prevalence of constipation, gastro-oesophageal reflux, obesity, food allergies Food aversions can occur, for example, some people with ASD are distressed by particular food textures	Ensure lifestyle information around diet/exercise is provided in an accessible format (e.g the person may understand pictures better than words) Consider the risk of osteoporosis in those with a restricted diet Consider referral to a dietitian with expertise in LD/ASD for those with food aversion
Respiratory: increased risk of aspiration, pneumonia, obstructive sleep apnoea	Consider a referral to a speech and language therapist with expertise in learning disability for a swallowing safety assessment Poor sleep can impact on behaviour during the day – consider referral to a sleep specialist
Neurological: increased prevalence of epilepsy, lower age of onset of dementia in people with a learning disability (e.g. Down's syndrome)	Seizures may be subtle and not readily observable Antiepilepsy medication can affect mood and behaviour – refer to neurology when this is suspected Consider dementia in those with a change in skills and refer for a specialist learning disability dementia assessment
Immunological: increased risk of immune system deficiency/dysfunction	Can experience frequent infections (e.g. ears, sinuses) – need to have a broad differential diagnosis
Mental illness	Mental illnesses, such as depression, are more common in people with ASD and LD than the general population, but can present atypically, requiring specialist assessment – consider referral to a learning disability psychiatrist

Box 12.9 Case vignette: Gordon – making reasonable adjustments in clinical care

Gordon's GP arranged to visit Gordon at home as Gordon would be more relaxed in a familiar environment. At home, Gordon was able to use symbols to indicate that his teeth hurt. The carers explained that Gordon is too anxious to tolerate going to the dentist or having his teeth brushed. The GP prescribed analgesia for likely dental pain and referred Gordon to the specialist dental service, who found that Gordon lacked capacity to consent to dental examination and treatment, and, together with the GP and Gordon's family and carers, decided examination and treatment under sedation was in his best interests.

Dental examination revealed Gordon had significant dental caries and required two extractions. Following recovery from his dental procedures, Gordon was happier, his appetite returned to normal, and he was no longer hitting himself in the face. The GP also referred Gordon to the local community LD team for support to reduce his distress around having his teeth brushed, and attending GP and dental appointments.

Box 12.10 Behaviour which challenges

- Denotes behaviour of such intensity, frequency or duration that it threatens the physical safety of the person or others, or restricts their access to community facilities
- Examples include:
  - physical aggression to self (e.g. biting or hitting self)
  - physical aggression to others (e.g. hitting, kicking, biting others)
  - causing destruction to the environment or property (e.g. throwing and breaking objects)

As with any concerns around behaviour (Box 12.7), underlying physical and mental health, and environmental/social factors, must be explored. Once these factors have been addressed, psychosocial interventions are key. These are underpinned by detailed analysis of the antecent, behaviour and consequences of the behaviour. From this, people supporting the individual learn how to modify triggers and consequences to diminish the occurrence of the behaviour.

Early implementation of psychosocial interventions is important to prevent challenging behaviours becoming entrenched, and to mitigate the effect on the individual and those supporting them (e.g. carer strain).

There are no licensed pharmacological treatments for behaviour which challenges in adults with ASD and LD. When psychosocial interventions are of limited effectiveness, or when the behaviour is associated with severe risks to the individual or to others, psychotropic medication can be considered to target specific symptoms (e.g. SSRIs to reduce anxiety) (Box 12.11).

When psychotropic medication is prescribed, effectiveness, side effects and the need for continuation or discontinuation should be reviewed regularly.

Box 12.11 Approach to behaviour which challenges in people with ASD and LD (adapted from National Institute for Health and Care Excellence guideline NG11 on Challenging Behaviour and Learning Disabilities, 2015)

1 Consider possible underlying causes: physical health, mental health, environmental/social factors
2 Offer a psychosocial intervention first, informed by functional analysis of the behaviour
3 Consider pharmacological interventions to target specific symptoms (e.g. anxiety), in addition to psychosocial interventions when there is limited response to psychosocial interventions alone
4 Consider pharmacological interventions alone when psychosocial interventions cannot be provided because of the severity of the behaviour that challenges

Box 12.12 Stopping Over-Medication of People with a learning disability, autism, or both (STOMP)

- In 2016, NHS England made the STOMP pledge to reduce the use of inappropriate psychotropic medication among people with ASD and/or LD
- The STOMP toolkit provides guidance on reducing and discontinuing psychotropic medication in primary care and general hospitals (see Further reading)

Psychotropic medication, autism and learning disability

Concerns about inappropriate psychotropic medication prescribing for people with ASD and/or LD have, in the UK, led to efforts to improve clinical practice in this area (Box 12.12).

Primary care clinicians are well-placed to identify people with ASD and/or LD inappropriately prescribed psychotropic medication, particularly those no longer under the care of secondary specialist services.

Annual health checks (Box 12.8) provide an opportunity for primary care clinicians to review psychotropic treatment response and side effects. When contemplating a reduction in psychotropic medication, primary care clinicians should consider referral to a learning disability psychiatrist.

Further reading

Equality Act 2010. London: The Stationery Office.

Heslop P, Blair PS, Fleming P, Hoghton M, Marriott A, Russ L. The Confidential Inquiry into premature deaths of people with intellectual disabilities in the UK: a population-based study. Lancet 2014; 383: 889–895.

Hirvikoski T, Mittendorfer-Rutz E, Boman M, Larsson H, Lichtenstein P, Bölte S.. Premature mortality in autism spectrum disorder. British Journal of Psychiatry 2016; 208: 232–238.

Mental Capacity Act. 2005. London: The Stationery Office.

National Institute for Health and Care Excellence (NICE). Challenging behaviour and learning disabilities: prevention and interventions for people with learning disabilities whose behaviour challenges. NICE guideline NG11. London: NICE, 2015. Available from: https://www.nice.org.uk/guidance/ng11. Accessed: 21 November 2018.

NHS England. Stopping Over-Medication of People with a learning disability, autism or both (STOMP): toolkit for reducing inappropriate psychotropic drugs in general practice and hospitals. Available from: https://www.england.nhs.uk/wp-content/uploads/2017/07/stomp-gp-prescribing-v17.pdf. Accessed: 21 November 2018.

Royal College of General Practitioners. Health checks for people with learning disabilities toolkit. Available from: http://www.rcgp.org.uk/clinical-and-research/resources/toolkits/health-check-toolkit.aspx. Accessed: 21 November 2018.

CHAPTER 13

Gender and Autism

Alison Stansfield, Padakkara Saju, Isabelle Gately, Kate Cooper, Derek Glidden, and Ruth Bevan

---

OVERVIEW

- Autistic people are over-represented in referrals to gender identity services.
- 'Sex' refers to the biological construct of a person based on their genital/body appearance.
- 'Gender' is a psychological, social and cultural construct.
- Gender dysphoria occurs when a person experiences distress because of a mismatch between their biological sex and gender identity.
- A complex set of biological and environmental factors contribute to an individual's gender identity.
- Using acceptable language is vital when interacting with the transgender community because of their vulnerability.
- Gender dysphoria amplifies autistic traits and this can account for some of the increased prevalence of autism in those with gender dysphoria.

There is increasing evidence that autistic people are over-represented in referrals to gender identity services.

Autistic people struggle with social interaction on a daily basis. Research shows they can also have altered self-representation (i.e. have problems thinking about and making sense of themselves). For some autistic persons, in addition to working out how they fit into a neurotypical world, issues of gender can also prove confusing. So how can we ensure that assessments untangle those people with gender dysphoria requiring treatment?

'Trans': what do you need to know?

The demarcation of sex as a biological construct and gender as a psychosocial construct is useful, but in many cultures sex, gender, gender role expression and sexual attraction and orientation get mixed up. The term 'construct' is used to denote a complex idea that may contain various conceptual elements which can often be, but are not always, considered as subjective rather than empirical.

Gender identity is one's internally felt and experienced sense of gender as a man, woman – or a combination of both sexes, or neither (agender).

Ultimately, gender identity is defined by oneself and this means a proliferation of terms, as people want to express their unique identity (Box 13.1).

Gender identity does not have to be fixed. For some people gender is experienced as fluid and changeable. Many people can experience a degree of gender dissonance.

Gender dysphoria – what is it?

Gender dysphoria is where there is a marked incongruence between gender identity and assigned sex or sexual characteristics and where this is associated with distress or discomfort. In this situation, an individual's functioning (social and occupational) can be significantly impaired and they may desire hormonal and/or surgical treatment to resolve the gender incongruence. Treatment is individualised, and is based on best practice guidelines.

Gender identity development and autism – what we know

A complex set of biological and environmental factors contribute to an individual's gender identity. Gender identity develops in the social world – a world that autistic people struggle to navigate. In typical development, children know their gender group by the age of 2.5–3 years. During development, gender norms are implicitly and explicitly taught to children through the behaviours of their caregivers and are reinforced by other children. Furthermore, children are likely to be bullied and ostracised by their peers if they transgress gender norms. This pressure to conform can reduce from adolescence to adulthood. Autistic children and young people are less attuned to the social world, and so may be less aware of such social norms and rules relating to gender, particularly in their early development.

The current literature has shown that there are high rates of gender variance in the autism community and that there are high rates of autism in those attending gender identity clinics.

Box 13.1 **Different terminologies in relation to gender identity**

Sex	The biological construct of a person based on their genital/body appearance
	Traditionally, people thought of sex as binary – male or female – but this is too simplistic
Gender	Gender is a psychological, social and cultural construct
Cisgender	If a person is happy in the gender they were assigned at birth they are described as a 'cis male' (biological male who is comfortable with the assigned gender of male) or 'cis female'
Trans/Transgender/Trans*	Terms to describe anyone who crosses the traditional gender boundaries of identity, role or expression
Non-binary	People whose identity and experience of gender falls outside of the gender binary of male and female
	Non-binary identities come in many forms (e.g. genderfluid, genderqueer, agender)

Box 13.2 **'Transgender' is an adjective**

'Transgender' is an adjective:
- It should not be used as a noun ('transgender') or a verb
- As with all adjectives, there should be a space between it and the word being described: e.g. '*A transgender woman*', '*A cisgender man*'

Box 13.3 **Different terminology**

While we would usually refer to 'transgender women' and 'transgender men', it is sometimes useful to make statements such as:
- All people **a**ssigned **m**ale **a**t **b**irth (AMAB)
- All people **a**ssigned **f**emale **a**t **b**irth (AFAB)

For example, 'AFAB people are at higher risk for breast cancer' is an easier way to state:
'Cisgender women, transgender men and non-binary individuals assigned female at birth are at higher risk for breast cancer'
AMAB and AFAB are more respectful synonyms of outdated terms like 'female-bodied' or 'biologically male'

Box 13.4 **Pronouns used by non-binary individuals**

They/them/their
Ze/hir/hir
Xe/xem/xir

Box 13.5 **The singular use of 'they'**

Consider the following dialogue:
A: I went to the doctor today
B: Really? What did they say?

Box 13.6 **Getting pronouns correct**

How to ask for pronouns
'What pronouns do you prefer?' (especially if the person you are addressing is known to be transgender)
If you are unsure whether a person might prefer non-standard pronouns, asking something like:
'How would you like me to refer to you?' can open up the conversation in a way that allows a transgender person to feel safe in disclosing that information

It is only when we use 'they' to refer to a specific person that it 'feels' unnatural. This is a matter of exposure and practice: as we get used to seeing it and using it, the more natural it becomes.

It is vital that the correct pronouns are used once they have been enquired about and ascertained (Box 13.6).

It is good practice to ask a transgender person for the name they would like to be used for them – and to use that name consistently. This may not always be the same name as that on their NHS record. It is worth bearing in mind that the cost of legally changing a name can be prohibitive and requires a ready income and a stable address, whilst transgender communities have high rates of homelessness and unemployment.

Using acceptable language

Using acceptable language is vital when interacting with the transgender community and clinicians should be aware of this (Boxes 13.2 and 13.3).

It is important to use the correct pronouns for non-binary individuals (Boxes 13.4 and 13.5), as they often use pronouns outside of 'he' and 'she'.

The use of 'they' as a singular pronoun can cause confusion as it first appears to be grammatically incorrect. In actual fact, we use 'they' to refer to an individual all the time when their gender is unknown.

Gender dysphoria and autism

Transgender health centres in the UK receive referrals for autistic people in the same way as for neurotypical people. However, the clinical history of gender dysphoria in someone with autism may not be typical (Box 13.7).

Providing transgender health care to those with autism can prove challenging for a number of reasons (Box 13.8), although this is not always the case. These difficulties can be magnified when there is limited knowledge of or training in autism and/or transgender health care respectively.

Box 13.7 **Different presentations of gender dysphoria in someone with autism**

- The early history of gender incongruency may be absent and/or overshadowed by autistic difficulties
- The awareness of their internal gender identity/experienced dysphoria in relation to their assigned gender at birth may be delayed until puberty or later
- They may describe exploration of their gender identity and gender role in gaming and in more online spaces
- They may describe a more cognitive description of their history of gender dysphoria with less verbally communicated emotional content
- A history of autistic arousal and/or 'meltdowns' in the presence of significant levels of gender dysphoria may be significant
- They may have difficulty with 'two-way gender recognition' – understanding that their own internal experience of their gender and the way others experience their gender may be different (i.e. others may not see them as male even though they see themselves as male')

Box 13.8 **Challenges to providing transgender health care to those with autism**

- Difficulties with two-way communication
- Difficulties with therapeutic alliance
- Difficulties with social function
- Co-morbid physical health problems
- Co-morbid mental health problems
- Geographical location
- Environmental factors
- Co-working and effective working with their family, professional and/or social network

There is no robust research on treatment outcomes for treating gender dysphoria in autistic people but some professionals feel that the outcomes are no worse than treating gender dysphoria in the neurotypical population. Treatment outcomes including hormonal treatment and gender affirming surgery have been robustly shown to be very good in the general population. Therefore autism is not, and should not be, a bar to transgender health care.

Coexistent intellectual disability, autism and gender variance

Individuals with autism and coexisting intellectual disability have similar experiences in regard to their gender identity (Figure 13.1). However, this area has a limited evidence base (Box 13.9).

Generalisations about people who have intellectual disability, autism and gender dysphoria cannot be made. The expectation that everyone presenting with gender dysphoria will give a similar and 'typical' history is unhelpful and potentially harmful. Having an intellectual disability and autism (or a coexisting mental health problem which should be managed appropriately) should not be a barrier to accessing help and support from appropriately trained

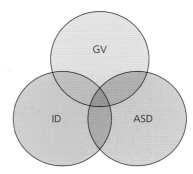

Figure 13.1 The overlap between autism (ASD), coexisting intellectual disability (ID) and gender variance (GV).

Box 13.9 **The presentation of gender variation in autistic people and intellectual disabilities**

- There is limited research in this area
- There is no specific evidence base or guidelines for this group
- Cognitive ability can influence presentation
- Individuals may display behaviours rather than make declarations about their gender
- Gender variation is unlikely to present in individuals who are non-verbal
- When present there may be more rigid views about gender role and sexuality
- Low self-esteem is an under-acknowledged issue which can lead some to want to make changes to their identity
- Role models can be influential, providing templates for gender. These are not always helpful

Box 13.10 **Tips for working with someone with intellectual disability and autism**

- Use appropriate language
- Check understanding
- Help the person to explore their gender identity by thinking and talking about it
- Exploration should not be confined to the clinic room, but continued outside, in their homes and communities (this may be met with barriers)
- Challenge rigid attitudes about gender identity especially gender roles and perhaps sexuality
- Discuss expectations frankly; they may be unrealistic and can lead to disappointment
- Consider the impact the environment has including a person's well-being and safety

teams and individuals (Box 13.10). Clinical experience suggests appropriate treatment can have positive outcomes.

Mental capacity and gender

The issue of capacity is often raised in relation to this topic. Mental capacity refers to being able to make your own decisions, but gender is not a decision to be made and therefore cannot be challenged under the auspices of capacity. However, aspects of treatment and social transition may require capacity assessments and best interest decisions.

Further reading

Bedard C, Zhang HL, Zucker KJ. Gender identity and sexual orientation in people with developmental disabilities. Sexuality and Disability 2010; 28: 165–175.

Bejerot S, Eriksson JM. Sexuality and gender role in autism spectrum disorder: a case–control study. PLoS One 2014; 9: 1.

Carver PR, Yunger JL, Perry DG. Gender identity and adjustment in middle childhood. Sex roles 2003; 49: 95–109.

De Vries A, Noens I, Cohen-Kettenis P, van Berckelaer-Onnes I, Doreleijers T. Autism spectrum disorders in gender dysphoric children and adolescents. Journal of Autism and Developmental Disorders 2010; 40: 930–936.

George R, Stokes MA. Gender identity and sexual orientation in autism spectrum disorder. Autism 2017; 22: 970–982.

Jones R, Wheelwright S, Farrell K, et al. Brief report: female-to-male transsexual people and autistic traits. Journal of Autism and Developmental Disorders 2012; 42: 301–306.

Kristensen Z, Broome M. Autistic traits in an Internet sample of gender variant UK adults. International Journal of Transgenderism 2015; 16: 234–245.

Maccoby EE. The Two Sexes: Growing Up Apart, Coming Together, Vol. 4. Harvard University Press, 1998

Pasterski V, Gilligan L, Curtis R. Traits of autism spectrum disorders in adults with gender dysphoria. Archives of Sexual Behavior 2014; 43: 387–393.

Royal College of Psychiatrists. CR181: Good practice guidelines for the assessment and treatment of adults with gender dysphoria. Avialable from: http://www.teni.ie/attachments/14767e01-a8de-4b90-9a19-8c2c50edf4e1.pdf. Accessed: 20 November 2018.

Skagerberg E, Di Ceglie D, Carmichael P. Brief report: autistic features in children and adolescents with gender dysphoria. Journal of Autism and Developmental Disorders 2015; 45: 2628–2632.

CHAPTER 14

Getting On With Life As an Adult After a Diagnosis

Frances Needham

OVERVIEW

- Following a diagnosis of autism, people can experience a number of emotions some of which are similar to those experienced during grief.
- In England, adults who have been diagnosed with autism can request an assessment by social services in relation to their needs.
- Students with autism can apply for disabled students allowances to assist with academic support.
- Adults with a diagnosis can request help in gaining employment through a referral to a disability employment advisor.
- Employees can request support with employment and reasonable adjustments.
- A health hospital passport can help when accessing health assessment and intervention.

Note: The information in this chapter in relation to available resources is specific to the UK (but will differ somewhat between England, Scotland, Wales and Northern Ireland) but may also be applicable to people living outside the UK.

Coping with a diagnosis

A diagnosis of autism can help a person to understand why they are the way they are; some describe this as a 'lightbulb moment'. It can also aid help family members, teachers, friends and employers to understand why the person thinks and behaves differently from other people, and this allows them to better support the affected individual. A diagnosis can also make it easier to identify coexisting conditions such as mental health issues and for this to be done earlier.

How people with autism cope following a diagnosis depends on their individual personalities and the support mechanisms around them.

Following a diagnosis of autism, people often feel a number of emotions: some feel relief, that they now have an explanation of why they are different from other people; others experience feelings typical of those who are grieving, such as shock or disbelief. Many adults and their carers feel angry that their difficulties were not recognised at school or by other professionals; others feel that the behaviours that they always thought were caused by their own personality no longer belong to them but to the diagnosis of autism (Box 14.1). It can take time for some to come to terms with the diagnosis, to see the way forward and to acknowledge that they are different from their peers (Box 14.2).

Post-diagnostic assessments

Many diagnostic services offer a follow-up appointment to provide adults who have been diagnosed with an opportunity to discuss their diagnosis in more detail and to provide information regarding local services. According to the Autism Act 2009, adults who have received a diagnosis should be offered an assessment of need by their local social services. (Carers are also entitled to an assessment.) The assessment should be carried out by someone who has had training in pertinent autism-related issues. The assessment does not automatically enable access to services, as many adults with autism do not require additional support or specialist services. However, it should be noted that even those with a high IQ can find some daily living activities difficult and require help with planning meals, shopping, budgeting as well as planning appointments. Keeping a copy of the diagnostic letter or report is essential as this can help with reasonable adjustments to be made for those who access further education or who are employed or for those applying for benefits.

Students

University students with a diagnosis of autism can apply for disabled students allowances. The diagnosis can allow academic-related support such as help with time management, work planning, structure, routine and examination arrangements. Some universities run support groups for students who have a diagnosis of autism. Quiet rooms, or spaces, for people with autism or mental health issues to access when they are feeling overwhelmed are available in some further and higher education establishments.

ABC of Autism, First Edition. Munib Haroon.
© 2019 John Wiley & Sons Ltd. Published 2019 by John Wiley & Sons Ltd.

Box 14.1 **Case vignette: John**

John is a 47-year-old man who came for assessment for autism. He was unsure as to whether he did have autism but had always felt different from other people. He had a number of obsessive interests such as collecting china egg cups from the age of 10 years and building Airfix models which he had kept but never played with. He could talk passionately about his interests to his family but had great difficulty in making small talk with people at work and preferred to sit in a corner of the office by himself at lunch time reading about his interests. His belongings on his desk were carefully laid out and he did not like these to be moved when his desk was cleaned. He always made lists of tasks he needed to accomplish throughout each day and stuck rigidly to these. Because of his lack of interaction with colleagues and difficulty with adjusting to changes in the workplace, John experienced a difficult work appraisal and did not achieve the promotion he had hoped for. John had always thought his behaviours and limited social interaction were part of his personality. John needed time to adjust to his diagnosis after finding out that other people with autism had intense interests and similar behaviours and these were not just his own idiosyncrasies. However, after receiving his diagnosis he was able to provide information about autism for his employers who provided advanced notice and preparation regarding changes in the workplace and he was able to talk to other employees about his diagnosis.

Box 14.2 **Case vignette: Jennie**

Jennie is a 35-year-old woman who had been encouraged to seek an assessment by her mental health nurse. Jennie had completed a masters degree in archaeology but had struggled with interviews and had not found herself suitable employment. She repeatedly stated that she did not think she had autism and was advised that she did not have to go through with the assessment but continued to attend appointments. Jennie had a habit of twiddling her hair for hours on end and she did not like to be touched. She would phone professionals repeatedly to explain that she could not have autism because of her intellectual ability. On being given a diagnosis of Asperger's syndrome she became very angry. Despite attending her follow-up appointment she would not accept her diagnosis. Six months later she contacted the service to say that after extensive research and reading she now recognised that she did have autism and after acknowledging her diagnosis on a job application was able to obtain an interview and was offered a job as an archaeologist.

Employment

Many adults with a diagnosis of autism continue to find it difficult to find employment, but some employers acknowledge that those with a diagnosis of autism have a great deal to offer in the workplace as they can be reliable, possess good time management skills and attention to detail, and perform to a very high standard, especially in areas related to their specialist skills. Despite this, about 20% of autistic adults, according to some estimates, are in full-time work and this figure has stayed relatively static for many years.

Persons with autism work in very many different areas including the arts and sciences; however, in order to flourish in some roles, a person with autism may need to have a specially adapted workplace, or role, as well as a sympathetic line manager. Under the Disability Discrimination Act, employers have to make reasonable adjustments for people who have a diagnosis of autism. This can include a quiet working space, the use of headphones to block out the noise in a busy office, adjustable lighting and help with communicating with other employees.

Support in obtaining employment is available through a referral to a disability employment advisor and local job centres can assist with this. The National Autistic Society provides fact sheets on their website for employers and employees.

Social activities

Adults with autism can often find themselves very isolated and may welcome the opportunity to meet other people through autism hubs, local support groups and special interest groups. Social media is also helpful for those people who find social interaction especially difficult. Some cinemas now provide autism friendly screenings with reduced sound, increased lighting, the opportunity to move around and with the film starting at the specified time without long series of adverts. Some theatres also provide special performances for people with autism. Walking groups, cycling clubs, running groups, tennis clubs and trampoline groups can provide opportunities to meet with others and for regular exercise which can help with anxiety management. It is felt that taking part in such pastimes can improve subjective and objective adult outcomes in those with autism.

Staying safe

Adults with autism can be very vulnerable and may not always have their needs recognised by others. For those who are able to go out alone, the use of an Autism Alert card, provided by the National Autistic Society, can help in times of difficulty and can be shown to police or health professionals who may not immediately understand why the person is having difficulty with communication or social interaction. Having an arrangement with regards to phoning a friend or relative on a regular basis, especially when out at night time, can help lower the risk to people who become easily overwhelmed. Various phone apps are available for people with autism to use in times of stress and anxiety; these can remind them of what to do and who to contact. The use of Telecare can also be useful for people who may put themselves at risk in the home environment.

Accommodation

Accommodation requirements vary from one individual to the next, and what works well at one point in time for a person may not work well when personal circumstances change. Individuals can obtain further advice specific to the part of the UK they live in from social services or their local housing authority.

Some adults with autism continue to live with family members on a permanent basis for many years. Estimates vary and are affected by different methodologies, geographies and timescales, but less than 20% of adults with autism, according to one review, live independently. In such circumstances, family members may be able to access a carer's assessment to address their needs. Whilst family members approach such an arrangement with great care and dedication, both parties sometimes require a break, and in this situation respite care can be very helpful.

Home support/Homecare involves having a care worker visit an individual's home on a regular basis. This can be funded by the individual/their family or by the council. This option can be useful for those who need help with personal care, housekeeping, nursing and companionship. It can take the form of sessions of varying length or be long term and run over 24 hours.

Residential care is a type of shared housing scheme where residents have support from staff (often round the clock) but are able to live relatively independent lives. Other options include supported living schemes, home-share schemes and supported lodging schemes.

Relationships

It is important to understand that the perception of people with autism being loners, who do not value contact, is often incorrect and that the many varied relationships of kith and kin, including friendships and more intimate relations, matter a great deal to persons on the autism spectrum (Figure 14.1). However, the difficulties associated with the core features of the condition – social communication and social interaction difficulties and other associated issues – can pose special challenges for those affected, and for their nearest and dearest. Despite these challenges, many autistic adults have partners and children and learn to manage their difficulties effectively. There are a wide range of books including some written by people who have autism which can prove useful resources for those who are affected and for those who have a relationship with them.

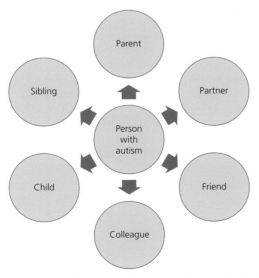

Figure 14.1 A person with autism can have many different relationships that are of great value to him/her – just like anybody else.

Health needs

People with autism can experience the same mental and physical illnesses as those in the general population, but they have a higher risk of some conditions and a well-documented increased mortality from suicide and epilepsy (see Chapter 15). Some people may be hyposensitive to pain but do not communicate their discomfort to other people so that when they do present with symptoms it is in a crisis situation. Admission to hospital can be very stressful for people with autism, because of their difficulties with communication and social interaction and hypersensitivity to noise. The My Hospital Passport, which can be downloaded free of charge from the National Autistic Society website, is a useful document as it can be completed and updated by the person with autism and their carer together. Copies can be given to GPs, dentists and other health professionals, and spare copies can be kept to be used if the person requires assessment in hospital. It is useful to keep a copy of a leaflet explaining what autism is along with it.

The environment

Specialists in the field of autism are becoming increasingly aware of the effect that the environment has on adults with autism, and it is well recognised that adjustments such as cream-painted walls, thick plain carpets and the use of natural or adjustable lighting can help. Avoiding the use of slatted blinds can reduce issues with light for some people. Having specific rooms for specific activities is also helpful for those who require predictability. Keeping things organised with specific things in specific places and avoiding clutter can help in reducing anxiety. For some people with severe disabilities, risks can be reduced by keeping electrical equipment in locked cabinets, whilst alarms on doors and gates can alert carers if people leave the house or garden.

People with autism often appreciate having something in their hands or pockets to fiddle with – such as stress balls or tangles – to reduce anxiety. Some people find moulding modelling clay comforting. Safe spaces for people to escape to, such as a garden with adequate fencing, can help when people are feeling overwhelmed. The use of paper towels instead of hand dryers is more helpful for people who are hypersensitive to noise. Being aware that some people find the use of strong disinfectants, cleaning materials, shampoos and perfumes difficult can reduce sensory difficulties. It is very important not to make too many changes to the environment at any one time – for example to an autistic person's immediate working space – and to explain any changes such as redecorating in advance. Organisations who have made changes to their environments to accommodate the needs of people with autism can apply for the National Autistic Society Autism Friendly Award.

Coping with sensory needs

People with autism can be hypersensitive or hyposensitive to noise, light, taste, textures and smells. They can also have difficulty with spatial awareness, balance and coordination.

The use of ear defenders or ear plugs can help those who are hypersensitive to noise; although care is required when using them near traffic. Earplugs and blackout curtains can help with sleep difficulties. Some people find the use of tinted lenses helpful if hypersensitive to light. Gradually introducing new tastes and textures can be helpful to those with restricted diets because of sensory issues.

Tactile issues can also create difficulty. People with autism sometimes strip off their clothing when they are extremely anxious as they can no longer tolerate the texture, whilst others can be very reluctant to change into different clothes. In this situation, ordering several items of the same garment that the person can tolerate can be helpful. Purchasing toiletries that do not have strong perfumes such as those for use by people with sensitive skin can be helpful in encouraging people to bathe or shower, and washing clothing in non-biological washing powders can reduce hypersensitivity.

Predictability

People with autism appreciate knowing what is going to happen in advance as this reduces anxiety. The use of calendars or diaries to remind people of events or appointments is helpful along with the use of apps on mobile phones. Individual timetables can be helpful for those people who also have learning disabilities. For those who prefer visual prompts, or for those who have difficulty with words, the use of symbols can be helpful when producing visual planners.

Communication and social interaction

To a person with autism the world can be a very confusing place and listening to conversations can sometimes feel as though people are speaking in a foreign language. People with autism require time to process what has been said and some people may need to repeat conversations to try to make sense of what they have heard. Carers and relatives can help by saying one thing at a time and using clear language without the use of words and phrases which have more than one meaning.

Some people with autism feel that they want to meet other people but have difficulty starting conversations. Memorising a list of conversation starters such as 'What have you been doing today?' and 'Have you been on holiday this year?' can be helpful in addition to participating in social skills training.

Written lists of instructions such as how to use the washing machine and other household equipment can promote independence. Easy to read recipes with photos or symbols can be helpful for people who have difficulty following the usual recipe books.

Christmas and other special occasions

Although many people enjoy special events such as Christmas, parties and family gatherings, for people with autism they can be very stressful. People with autism often cannot cope with lots of noise and having to interact with a room full of people and will try to avoid such events. Therefore special events have to be planned very carefully, well in advance, with opportunities to escape from the celebrations if required. The use of Social Stories invented by Carol Gray can help adults with learning disabilities and autism to prepare for special events such as moving house, going on holiday or family occasions such as a wedding or to gain social skills in particular situations. Ensuring that a separate room is available to escape to and the use of headphones and an iPad can all be helpful.

Driving

According to one estimate, only 27% of people with autism also have a driving licence. Whilst having autism, per se, is not a barrier to being able to drive, it is a condition that could affect driving – for example, because of coexisting epilepsy. In the UK, in such instances, it is important for an individual to inform the Driver and Vehicle Licensing Agency (DVLA).

Further reading

Atwood T, Evans C, Lesko A, eds. Been there. Done That. TRY THIS! An Aspie's Guide to Life on Earth. London: Jessica Kingsley, 2014.

Autism Act 2009. Available from: http://www.legislation.gov.uk/ukpga/2009/15/contents. Accessed: 21 November 2018.

Booth J. Autism in the work place. Trades Union Congress, 2014. Available from: https://www.tuc.org.uk/sites/default/files/Autism.pdf. Accessed: 21 November 2018.

Gray C. The New Social Story Book. Future Horizons, 2010.

Henninger N, Taylor J. Outcomes in adults with autism spectrum disorder: a historical perspective. Autism 2012; 17: 103–116.

National Autistic Society. www.autism.org.uk/

National Autistic Society. The autism employment gap: too much information in the workplace. NAS, 2016.

National Institute for Health and Clinical Excellence. Autism spectrum guidance in adults: diagnosis and management. NICE Guideline CG142. London: NICE, 2012 (updated 2016). Available from: https://www.nice.org.uk/guidance/cg142. Accessed: 21 November 2018.

Think Autism. Fulfilling and rewarding lives, the strategy for adults with autism in England: an update. Available from: https://www.gov.uk/government/uploads/system/uploads/attachment_data/file/299866/Autism_Strategy.pdf. Accessed: 21 November 2018.

CHAPTER 15

Mortality and Autism

Alwyn Kam

OVERVIEW

- Autism is associated with a reduced lifespan.
- On average, autistic people die 16 years earlier than the general population, whilst individuals who also have a learning disability die on average 30 years earlier.
- There is an increased risk of death from neurological disease (especially epilepsy) in people with autism and learning disabilities (intellectual disabilities), and suicide in people with autism without a learning disability.
- Appropriate monitoring and management of coexisting conditions in individuals with autism is important throughout life.

There is growing evidence to show that autism is associated with a reduced lifespan and a range of health problems because of combined biological, social, environmental and health care/provision factors.

Older research studies and mortality

Older studies in children with autism (Boxes 15.1 and 15.2) have pointed towards an increase in mortality from several causes: seizures, and accidents – such as suffocation and drowning. They have suggested a higher mortality from respiratory disease in those with severe learning disabilities. Whilst higher mortality rates were found in children with severe learning disabilities, life expectancy was reduced even for children with milder co-morbid conditions (e.g. mild learning disabilities).

A number of older studies reported that autistic adults were at increased risk of dying at an earlier age than those without autism. However, until recently, most studies have been too small to examine other factors in detail.

Recent studies on mortality

Two of the most recent studies are worth examining in greater detail.

Schendel et al. (2015) identified and followed a cohort of over 20 000 Danish children with autism born between 1980 and 2010

through to 2013. The overall adjusted mortality risk (hazard ratio) of 2.0 (95% CI 1.5–2.8) was similar to previous studies. The factor most strongly associated with a raised mortality in autistic people was the presence of co-morbid neurological disorders (adjusted mortality risk of 7.6; 95% CI 4.4–13.2). In addition, the presence of mental and/or behavioural disorders in those with autism was associated with an increased mortality (adjusted mortality risk = 2.6; 95% CI 1.8–3.8).

There was a 4.6-fold increased risk of death from intentional self-harm and the majority of these persons had known mental and/or behavioural co-morbid conditions. The authors found that overall mortality was quite rare in children and young adults (affecting only 0.3% of those with autism) and that the risk of death among children under 18 was not statistically significantly raised.

The Swedish study carried out by Hirvikoski et al. (2016) examined the records from Sweden's national registers of 27 122 people diagnosed with autism and analysed life expectancy, the main causes of death, and the influences of factors such as learning disabilities and sex.

This study divided those with autism into two groups: low-functioning autism, which included adults with autism with a learning disability (i.e. they had an IQ below 70); and high-functioning autism, which included adults with autism who had average or above average intelligence (they had an IQ of 70 or above).

Overall, those with autism in this study had increased odds (2.56-fold) of mortality compared to people who were not autistic (matched population controls). The increased mortality was seen across most causes, apart from infections. In autistic people with learning disabilities this included a significantly increased risk of dying from neurological disease (including epilepsy), whilst those without learning disabilities were at an increased risk of death by suicide (Figure 15.1).

Overall, people with low-functioning autism had more than a fivefold increase in the odds of mortality compared to matched population controls, whilst those with high functioning autism had more than a twofold increase in the odds of mortality compared to matched population controls.

ABC of Autism, First Edition. Munib Haroon.
© 2019 John Wiley & Sons Ltd. Published 2019 by John Wiley & Sons Ltd.

Box 15.1 **Terminology used in this chapter**

Learning disabilities Also termed 'intellectual disabilities'. Individuals with a learning disability have an IQ of less than 70 and loss of adaptive social functioning

Autism This term is used in this chapter to describe autism and other autism spectrum disorders, including Asperger's syndrome

Low-functioning autism People with autism and a learning disability

High-functioning autism People with autism who do not have a learning disability

Box 15.2 **A summary of key studies in autism and mortality**

Shavelle et al. (2001) This study followed a cohort of 13 111 children of all IQ in California, USA between 1983 and 1997. The calculated mortality risk ratio was **2.4** for children with autism. This cohort was re-examined in 2006 over the follow-up period 1998–2002, the risk ratio was **2.6**

Mouridsen et al. (2008) This cohort study in Denmark followed-up 340 people (including children) between 1960 and 2006. Autistic people had a mortality risk ratio of **1.9**. This study found a higher mortality risk in females but no significant difference in people with learning disabilities

Schendel et al. (2015) A large cohort of 20 492 children with autism were followed up in Denmark from 1980 to 2013. This study calculated an overall adjusted mortality risk (hazard ratio) of **2.0** for those with autism

Hirvikoski et al (2016) This case–control study from Sweden looked at 27 122 people with autism who were diagnosed between 1987 and 2009. They looked at the risk from different causes of death, but the overall risk ratio for mortality for people with autism was **2.56**

Sex differences

Schendel et al. (2015) found that females with autism had a higher relative risk of death than males.

Hirvikovski et al. found that mortality was raised in both genders compared to the general population but that the risk was greatest in those with low-functioning autism. Females with low-functioning autism in particular were found to have 8.5-fold increased odds of mortality compared to females without autism (Table 15.1). The cause of death was associated with gender, with a greater mortality from diseases of the nervous and circulatory system in males, whilst diseases of the endocrine system and those from congenital malformations and suicide were associated with more deaths in women.

Life expectancy

Hirvikoski et al. found that the average age of death for a person with autism was 54 years, compared to 70 years for matched controls. In contrast to earlier studies, people with low-functioning

Table 15.1 Comparison of male and female mortality risk in two large studies.

Study		Males	Females
Hirvikovski et al. (2016)	Low-functioning autism	Odds ratio 4.88 (95% CI 4.02–5.93)	Odds ratio 8.52 (95% CI 6.55–11.08)
	High-functioning autism	Odds ratio 2.49 (95% CI 2.22–2.8)	Odds ratio 1.88 (95% CI 1.65–2.14)
	Total	Odds ratio 2.87 (95% CI 2.6–3.16)	Odds ratio 2.24 (95% CI 1.99–2.51)
Schendel et al. (2015)		Adjusted hazard ratio 1.8 (95% CI 1.2–2.6)	Adjusted hazard ratio 3.5 (95% CI 1.7–7.0)

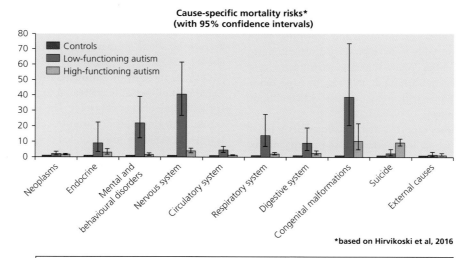

Cause-specific mortality risks*
(with 95% confidence intervals)

Controls
Low-functioning autism
High-functioning autism

Neoplasms, Endocrine, Mental and behavioural disorders, Nervous system, Circulatory system, Respiratory system, Digestive system, Congenital malformations, Suicide, External causes

*based on Hirvikoski et al, 2016

Low-functioning autism: There was a higher risk of death due to different categories of disorders including congenital malformations, mental health and behavioural conditions, and neurological and respiratory disorders.

High-functioning autism: There was a statistically highly significant difference in mortality in suicide as a cause of death.

Figure 15.1 Cause-specific mortality risks and significant findings (based on Hirvikovski et al. 2016).

autism were found, on average, to die before the age of 40 years. This suggests that, on average, autistic people appear to have a life expectancy 16 years shorter than the general population, and individuals who have a learning disability die 30 years earlier (Hirvikoski et al. 2016).

Causes of increased mortality in autism

Research into mortality rates have consistently shown an overall twofold increase (at least) in the odds of death in people with autism compared to the general population. By their nature, population studies look at associations (e.g. between having autism and dying early) but cannot prove what is causing those differences (causation). An added complication is that individuals with autism are a heterogeneous group; there are lots of other factors including the presence or absence of associated co-morbidities, like mental health conditions and epilepsy, to take into account (Boxes 15.3 and 15.4).

At present it seems reasonable to speculate that there are likely to be a number of underlying reasons that explain why autistic people might be more prone to health problems. Broadly speaking, these include biological, social, environmental and health care/provision factors – and these may well interact with each other (Figure 15.2).

Box 15.3 **Epilepsy and autism**

- Seizures are a significant concern and are the most prevalent neurological disorder associated with autism. While 1–2% of children in the general population develop epilepsy, the prevalence of epilepsy in autism is much higher with estimates of 5–38%. A range of seizure types are seen in individuals with autism and epilepsy, rather than any single epilepsy or seizure type
- Some people with autism develop seizures in childhood, but others might develop them in puberty or even in adulthood. The prevalence of seizures with age is not well studied, but recent findings suggest the risk of seizure remains high into adulthood
- Seizures are associated with increased mortality and morbidity in individuals with autism, and certain clinical subgroups have a higher risk for developing epilepsy, for example individuals with

co-morbid learning disabilities, genetic abnormalities and/or brain malformations
- Specific genetic and metabolic syndromes are associated with both autism and seizures, although in many cases the cause of the seizures remains unknown even after extensive investigations. Many of these investigations would likely be conducted in childhood. Some of the genetic disorders include fragile X syndrome, tuberous sclerosis and Prader–Willi syndrome, and metabolic syndromes include mitochondrial dysfunction and cerebral folate deficiency
- A NICE (National Institute for Health and Care Excellence) Evidence Update in 2014 looked at research on epilepsy and autism and emphasised the need for appropriate monitoring and management of coexisting conditions in adults with autism, particularly those with epilepsy

---

Box 15.4 **Suicide and autism**

Hirvikoski et al. (2016) found that the risk of death due to suicide was greatly increased in people with high-functioning autism. In general, such individuals often present with coexisting mental health disorders, but because of their greater intellectual ability they may attract less support for their difficulties, especially if their autism is unrecognised. People with autism often have difficulties in social interaction and communication and these can prevent them from seeking and receiving help and treatment. Appropriate service planning to manage risks in this group is therefore recommended.

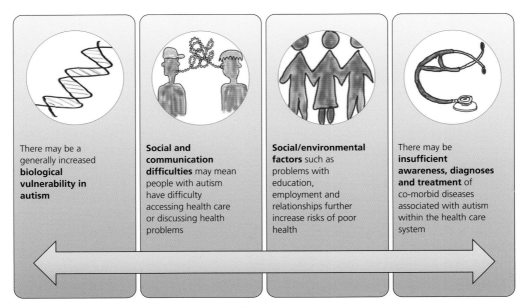

There may be a generally increased **biological vulnerability in autism**

Social and communication difficulties may mean people with autism have difficulty accessing health care or discussing health problems

Social/environmental factors such as problems with education, employment and relationships further increase risks of poor health

There may be **insufficient awareness, diagnoses and treatment** of co-morbid diseases associated with autism within the health care system

Figure 15.2 Common factors that may contribute to the increased mortality rates in autism.

Future directions

Despite the growing evidence base to show that autism is associated with a reduced lifespan, there is a limited understanding of how the different factors responsible for this (biological, social and environmental and health provision) interact with each other.

There is also a growing body of evidence showing how autism in a child may be linked to maternal mortality (the mothers of children with autism) because of cancer and psychiatric disease and this is an important area for future research.

Further work is required to address these topics, but there are several barriers to overcome when conducting such research. These include the 'capture' of a proper representative population of people across the entire spectrum with a reliable diagnosis, and who can then be followed up over many years. There is also the limitation in being able to show causation in association studies.

Nevertheless, the clear association between autism and mortality calls for raised awareness of this important topic. A better appreciation amongst society at large may allow for funding to be adequately directed towards research into this topic. It is also important that all professionals (and carers) who come into contact with persons with autism are aware of the associated mortality and health risks. It is important that a diagnosis of autism is not viewed as just 'a label' but also as a marker that an affected individual could be at risk of other life-limiting conditions.

Further reading

Autistica. 2016. Personal tragedies, public crisis. Available from: www.autistica.org.uk/wp-content/uploads/2016/03/Personal-tragedies-public-crisis.pdf. Accessed: 22 November 2018.

Cassidy S, Bradley P, Robinson J, Allison C, McHugh M, Baron-Cohen S. Suicidal ideation and suicide plans or attempts in adults with Asperger's syndrome attending a specialist diagnostic clinic: a clinical cohort study. Lancet Psychiatry 2014; 1: 142–147. doi: 10.1016/S2215-0366(14)70248-2.

Emerson E, Hatton C, Hastings R, Felce D, McCulloch A, Swift P. The health of people with autistic spectrum disorders. Tizard Learning Disability Review 2011; 16: 36–44.

Fairthorne JC, de Klerk NH, Leonard HM, Whitehouse AJO. Mothers of children with autism have different rates of cancer according to the presence of intellectual disability in their child. Journal of Autism and Developmental Disorders 2016; 46: 3106–3114.

Fairthorne JC, Hammond G, Bourke J, Jacoby P, Leonard H. Early mortality and primary causes of death in mothers of children with intellectual disability or autism spectrum disorder: a retrospective cohort study. PLoS One 2014; 9: e113430. doi:10.1371/journal.pone.0113430.

Hirvikoski T, Mittendorfer-Rutz E, Boman M, Larsson H, Lichtenstein P, Bölte S. Premature mortality in autism spectrum disorder. British Journal of Psychiatry 2016; 208: 232–238.

Mouridsen SE, Bronnum-Hansen H, Rich B, Isager T. Mortality and causes of death in autism spectrum disorders: an update. Autism 2008; 12: 403–414.

National Institute for Health and Care Excellence. Autism in adults: evidence update May 2014: a summary of selected new evidence relevant to NICE clinical guideline 142 'Autism: recognition, referral, diagnosis and management of adults on the autism spectrum' (2012). London: NICE, 2014. Available from: https://arms.evidence.nhs.uk/resources/hub/1035112/attachment. Accessed: 22 November 2018.

Schendel DE, Overgaard M, Christensen J, et al. Association of psychiatric and neurologic comorbidity with mortality among persons with autism spectrum disorder in a Danish population. JAMA Pediatrics 2016; 170: 243–250. doi:10.1001/jamapediatrics.2015.3935.

Takara K, Kondo T. Comorbid atypical autistic traits as a potential risk factor for suicide attempts among adult depressed patients: a case–control study. Annals of General Psychiatry 2014; 13: 1–8.

CHAPTER 16

Interventions for Autism in Children and Adults

Munib Haroon

OVERVIEW

- Pharmacological and non-pharmacological interventions do not 'cure' the core features of autism.
- Interventions for autism should be safe, timely, effective, efficient, equitable and patient-centred.
- Pharmacological interventions should be considered as adjuncts to behaviourally based and/or non-pharmacological interventions.

Questions about interventions, treatment and cures are common following the diagnosis of autism in a child, young person or adult. Whilst there are no shortages of interventions, none are curative or able to remove the core features of the condition.

Some interventions are based on sound, sensible and practical considerations underpinned by an understanding of the difficulties seen in autism spectrum disorder, but they may lack a firm evidence base as to their effectiveness.

High quality interventions

The Institute of Medicine in the USA published a report in 2001 in which they identified six dimensions relating to quality care: safety, timeliness, effectiveness, efficiency, equitability and patient-centredness (Figure 16.1). Interventions for autism, whether they are pharmacological or non-pharmacological, indeed any aspect of health care should aim to reflect these parameters.

Evidence based medicine

Where it exists, evidence about specific interventions for autism and how they address the different dimensions of good quality care can come from a number of different types of study or sources (Figure 16.2). Clinical guidelines, such as those issued in the UK by NICE and SIGN and which make recommendations on the basis of available evidence may draw their findings from a hierarchy of clinical studies. Although, sometimes, where research evidence is not available, recommendations are made on the basis of expert opinion. Expert opinion can either be based on the experience of a Guideline Development Group, using informal consensus processes, or be developed explicitly using formal consensus methodologies such as Delphi Panels.

Non-pharmacological interventions in children

These range from the simple to the complex; from interventions that can be put into place by parents to those that require ongoing support from professionals (Box 16.1). Not every type of intervention will be easily available, because of care commissioning arrangements, or worthwhile – when assessed for being of 'high quality'. Occasionally, parents will inquire about whether a particular programme or therapy can be paid for privately. In these circumstances it is important to be realistic and acknowledge the limited evidence for many interventions so that parents only commit to costly programmes once they are aware of the potential outcomes.

The terms used to describe interventions in the literature can often be generalised. For example, the term 'parent mediated interventions' can be used to describe a variety of programmes with different types of individual interventions administered for differing durations and frequencies. In addition, studies measure different outcomes, or use different tools, on different subsets of children with autism. This clinical and methodological heterogeneity can make it difficult to appraise the literature and come up with generalised 'broad-brush' recommendations. Where interventions have been shown to lead to improved outcomes it is then also crucial to ask how long the improvement lasts for: an ideal intervention would offer permanent, or at least long-lasting benefits.

For example, a recent Cochrane review looking at Early Intensive Behavioural Intervention found and analysed five studies noting weak evidence for improved outcomes in behaviour and language after two years of treatment and no improvements in the core traits of autism. On the other hand, a study looking at parent-mediated social communication therapy found that almost six years after an original randomised controlled trial had been carried out, children continued to show long-term symptom reduction.

ABC of Autism, First Edition. Munib Haroon.
© 2019 John Wiley & Sons Ltd. Published 2019 by John Wiley & Sons Ltd.

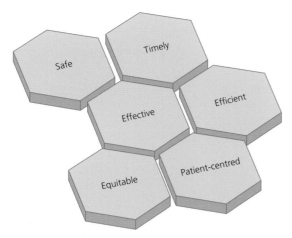

Figure 16.1 The six dimensions of high quality care.

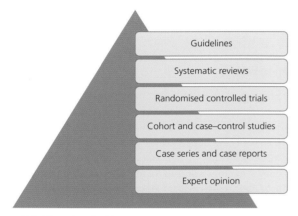

Figure 16.2 Hierarchy of evidence.

Box 16.1 **Behavioural interventions. Guidance issued by SIGN in 2016 stated that those indicated with ** *should* be considered for those with autism, whilst those indicated with * *may* be considered or *may* benefit those with autism. General recommendations were not made for other interventions where benefits were small (e.g. Social Stories) or where study quality made the framing of clear recommendations difficult.**

- Parent mediated interventions**
- Parents and clinician led interventions
- Visual supports
- Picture Exchange Communication System (PECS)**
- Environmental visual supports**
- Social skill groups**
- Computer based interventions**
- Early Intensive Behavioural Intervention
- Support from staff trained in Applied Behavioural Analysis technology**
- Treatment and Education of Autistic and related Communication handicapped Children (TEACCH)
- Social Stories
- Cognitive behavioural therapy*
- Auditory Integration Training
- Sensory Integration Training and occupational therapy*
- Music therapy
- Behavioural therapy for sleep**

As a general rule, it is important to consider behavioural interventions before pharmacological ones and to view pharmacological therapies not in isolation but as part of a package of care. As with pharmacological therapy, complex behavioural interventions should be administered by, or be led by, people with the necessary experience.

The evidence base for such interventions is rapidly evolving and may lead to the modifications of current recommendations made by national bodies like NICE and SIGN.

Pharmacological interventions in children

Medication is not curative and has not been shown to improve the core features of autism on the basis of long-term trials. As such, it should be used for managing associated psychiatric and neurodevelopmental co-morbidities, or for addressing specific and severe behaviours on a short to medium term basis, or for treating coexisting medical conditions such as epilepsy. Medication should not be used in isolation, but instead, when required, should form part of a wider package of care.

The right *medication*, at the right *time*, for the right *child*, by the right *person*

Before commencing medication it is important assess what condition or symptoms are being targeted and thus choose an appropriate drug (right *medication*). The child should be assessed not only in terms of their clinical presentation, but also assessed with respect to their wider circumstances – including those at school and at home – with the aim of seeing if modifications can be made to these areas first (right *time*). It is important to balance the risks with the benefits for medication, taking into account the child's other preexisting medical history (right *child*), and to have ensured that these issues are discussed and understood by the child/patient and carers and to define, as a baseline, which target features the treatment is supposed to address. There should then be a plan for how a child or young person will be monitored and how medication will be managed. Medication should be prescribed by those competent to do so (right *person*) and with reference to appropriate guidance such as the *British National Formulary (BNF)*. Some medications that can be useful are described in Table 16.1.

Non-pharmacological interventions for adults

There are a number of interventions that are available to support adults with autism. Such interventions are aimed at addressing a wide range of areas including: adaptive behaviours, communication, psychiatric co-morbidities, activities of daily living, employment and relationships.

However, many have been developed for children and young people, and so the evidence for their efficacy in adults is limited. Making recommendations in adults is further hampered where studies are small in scale or of low quality, and often clinical decisions have to be made on the basis of unclear or inconsistent evidence or on the basis of expert opinion.

Certainly, there seems to be some evidence to support the use of certain types of social skills programmes, behavioural interventions,

Table 16.1 Medications that can be used in patients with autism for specific indications.

Second generation antipsychotics e.g. aripiprazole	Can help in the short term (8 weeks) to reduce irritability and hyperactivity. Associated with significant side effects which prescribers should be aware of and communicate to carers/patients. Effectiveness should be reviewed after 3–4 weeks and medication stopped at 6 weeks if not effective Should not be used to manage the core features of autism
Medication for ADHD Methylphenidate	Medication for ADHD can be very effective and there is evidence to support the use of methylphenidate in children with ADHD-type symptoms and autism although it is limited The evidence for treating children and young persons with other drugs used to treat ADHD is less well-founded and should be considered with reference to national guidance, and the *BNF* by those experienced with their use
Antidepressants Selective serotonin reuptake inhibitors	Useful in children and young persons with coexisting conditions such as depression
Melatonin	To help with sleep alongside a consistent bedtime routine and sleep hygiene. This can be considered in children and young persons where there has been an insufficient improvement after behavioural interventions. Medication should be commenced in consultation with a paediatrician or psychiatrist with the relevant expertise and its use should be appropriately monitored

and also cognitive behavioural therapy in individuals with autism who have a condition such as anxiety or depression, where such therapy would be offered in an individual without autism (although such therapy may have to be adapted to individuals with autism, given their core difficulties with social communication and social interaction).

All such interventions should be delivered by those who are trained in their use, and should be accompanied by monitoring to see if the intervention achieves a change in desired target behaviour and to check for any adverse outcomes.

Pharmacological interventions in adults

Much of what was said about medication in children applies to adults. There is limited evidence to support the use of a wide range of medications for the treatment of specific symptoms in adults with autism. However, this should not stop them from being used – by those trained in their use – to treat coexisting conditions in adults who also happen to have autism. It is on this basis that medications such as anxiolytics, antidepressants, melatonin and drugs for treating ADHD should be used.

Antipsychotic medication use in ASD is supported by national guidance on the basis of a small number of trials (including two open label trials, and studies on adults with intellectual disabilities whose findings have been extrapolated to adults with autism) with the stipulation that it is not to address the core features of autism but for challenging behaviour where behavioural interventions have not worked. Efficacy should be reviewed at 3–4 weeks and medication stopped if there is no effect at 6 weeks.

Further reading

Institute of Medicine. Crossing the Quality Chasm: A New Health System for the 21st Century. Committee on Quality of Health Care in America. Institute of Medicine. Washington, DC: National Academies Press, 2001.

Pickles A, LeCouteur A, Leadbitter K, et al. Parent-mediated social communication therapy for young children with autism (PACT): long term follow-up of a randomised controlled trial. Lancet 2016; 388: 2501–2509.

Reichow B, Hume K, Barton EE, Boyd BA. Early intensive behavioral intervention (EIBI) for young children with autism spectrum disorders (ASD). Cochrane Database of Systematic Reviews 2018; 5: CD009260. doi:10.1002/14651858.CD009260.pub3.

Scottish Intercollegiate Guidelines Network (SIGN). SIGN 145: assessment, diagnosis and interventions for autism spectrum disorders. Edinburgh: SIGN, 2016. Available from: https://www.sign.ac.uk/assets/sign145.pdf. Accessed: 15 November 2018.

Index

ABC of autism. Locators in *italics* refer to figures and boxes.

ABC of Autism, First Edition. Munib Haroon.
© 2019 John Wiley & Sons Ltd. Published 2019 by John Wiley & Sons Ltd.

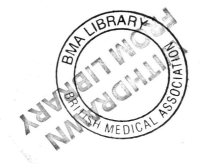